the **Do's** & **Don'ts**
of Hypoglycemia

AN EVERYDAY GUIDE TO LOW BLOOD SUGAR
TOO OFTEN MISUNDERSTOOD AND MISDIAGNOSED!

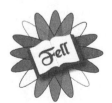

Frederick Fell Publishers, Inc
2131 Hollywood Blvd., Suite 305
Hollywood, Fl 33020
www.Fellpub.com
email: Fellpub@aol.com

Frederick Fell Publishers, Inc
2131 Hollywood Blvd., Suite 305
Hollywood, Fl 33020

This publication is designed to provide accurate and authoritative information in regard to the subject matter covered. It is sold with the understanding that the publisher is not engaged in rendering legal, medical, accounting, or other professional services. If legal advice or other assistance is required, the services of a competent professional person should be sought. From a Declaration of Principles jointly adopted by a Committee of the American Bar Association and a Committee of Publishers.

Printed in the United States of America.

14 13 12 11 10 9 8 7 6 5 4 3 2 1

Library of Congress Cataloging-in-Publication Data

Ruggiero, Roberta
 The Do's & Don'ts of Hypoglycemia : an everyday guide to low blood sugar : too often misunderstood and misdiagnosed! / by Roberta Ruggiero.
    p. cm.
 ISBN 978-0-88391-809-8 (pbk. : alk. paper)
 1. Hypoglycemia--Popular works. 2. Hypoglycemia--Diet therapy--Recipes.
3. Cookbooks. I. Title.

 RC662.2R84 2011
 616.4'660654--dc23
                          2011029971

For information about special discounts for bulk purchases, please contact Frederick Fell Special Sales at fellpub@aol.com or call 945-455-4243.

ISBN: 978-0-88391-809-8
ePUB: 978-0-88391-391-8

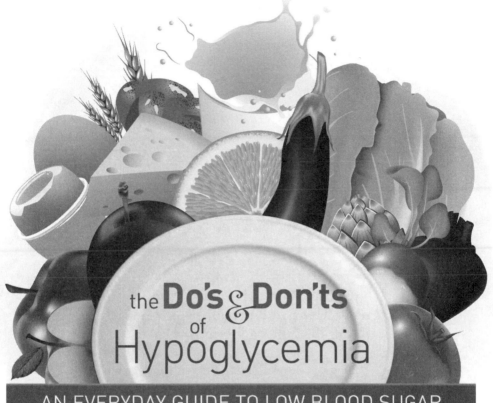

the **Do's** & **Don'ts**
of
Hypoglycemia

AN EVERYDAY GUIDE TO LOW BLOOD SUGAR
TOO OFTEN MISUNDERSTOOD AND MISDIAGNOSED!

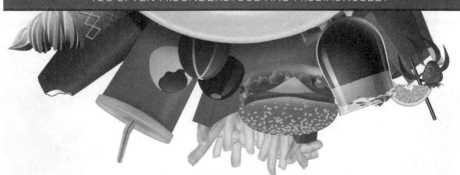

ROBERTA RUGGIERO
President and Founder of The Hypoglycemia Support Foundation, Inc.

" *Many books promise to cure your health problems, few deliver. Roberta Ruggiero understands the challenges of hypoglycemia from personal experience. She offers practical solutions in her book that are clear and compassionate. If you have been diagnosed with hypoglycemia, get this book. It could save your life.* "

— **Ken Nochimson, Executive Producer Public Television Program, Sweet Revenge: Turning the Tables on Processed Food**

WORDS OF ENDORSEMENT FROM...

"*The Do's and Don'ts of Low Blood Sugar* was chosen among the top best lay medical books because it covers a subject of potential interest to public library patrons in a responsible, easily understood way...A worthwhile edition to a public library collection."

—American Library Journal

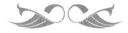

"*The Do's and Don'ts of Low Blood Sugar* has been endorsed in our programs. Only those books that are felt to be truly outstanding selections are incorporated into our programming. It's always a personal pleasure to encounter and recommend good, conscientious work to our audience."

—The Midwest Book Review
Oregon, Wisconsin

"You've done a superb job after years of both personal and intellectual research on this topic. Thank you for helping so many people who will benefit from your experiences and clear writing."

—Jeffrey S. Bland, Ph.D.
Gig Harbor, Washington

"Congratulations on a great book that really brings the whole question of low blood sugar into an easy to read, understandable form. You certainly answer every conceivable question that a patient is likely to ask, and I wish you every success."

—Robert Buist, Ph.D.

Sydney, Australia

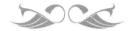

"I appreciate having received your book. The focus for me was the chapter which you discussed the approach to a positive attitude. I love the way you formulated your concepts and am happy for you that the book is in print."

—Leonard A. Wisneski, M.D., F.A.C.P.

Bethesda, Maryland

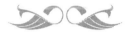

"My first suggestion to a hypoglycemic patient is to read your book. Education and understanding of hypoglycemia, or LBS, is probably the single most important thing that one can do to deal with this condition, and your book is a great place to start."

—Douglas M. Baird, D.O., P.A.

Tampa, Florida

"Roberta's book is an important addition to anyone's medical library. She helps the reader understand the complexities surrounding the under diagnosed epidemic of reactive hypoglycemia. Individuals after reading this book will recognize the symptoms associated with this condition and gain the tools needed to successful achieve better health. Because of her critical insights and the wisdom she shares from her journey, Roberta's book is a must read."

—Keith Berkowitz, M.D.

New York, New York

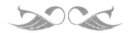

"Your latest book on low blood sugar is FANTASTIC! You have successfully distilled the essence of the subject for those that suffer from the often misdiagnosed and misunderstood condition of hypoglycemia. The information on diet, vitamins and exercise could easily be followed by anyone who is seeking health or wants to maintain their health."

—Leo B. Stouder, B.S., D.C., D.N.B.C.E.

Hollywood, Florida

"As I began to read your book, I couldn't help but feel that I was reading my own story with all the frustrations and fears that you experienced. I would also like to say thanks for all your time and effort you put forth in getting this book published and The Hypoglycemia Support Foundation started."

—Madison, Wisconsin

"The book was a tremendous lift to my spirits and renewed my courage to keep up the pace on the road to recovery. I wish that every person who has hypoglycemia or is suffering the symptoms and doesn't know the cause could read this book. It is a great support!"

—**Selma**
North Carolina

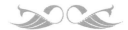

"I believe your book, *The Do's and Don'ts of Low Blood Sugar*, could be the most helpful thing a newly diagnosed hypoglycemic could read. Its simplicity of style makes it an excellent first choice. How I wish it had been available to me in 1980."

—**Del City, Oklahoma**

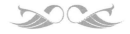

"I have just finished reading your book, *The Do's and Don'ts of Low Blood Sugar*, which I picked up at the library. It is the most informative book I have found to date."

—**East Lyme, Connecticut**

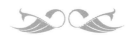

"My doctor has informed me that I am 'borderline diabetic' and he has recommended that I read the book titled *The Do's and Don'ts of Low Blood Sugar*.

—**Summerland Key, Florida**

"I have scoured bookstores and health food stores and every place else I could think of for information. I was quite discouraged until yesterday when I went to the library. I found a copy of your *Do's and Don'ts of Low Blood Sugar*. I was thrilled with all of the information you included in this book. From my own experience I know how much work must have been involved in gathering it. I finally feel like my husband and I will be able to get a handle on our situation and keep his condition in check."

—Houston, Texas

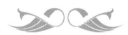

"Your book *The Do's and Don'ts of Low Blood Sugar* was a life saver. After more than 15 years I have finally found my cure: a simple diet!"

—Poland, Ohio

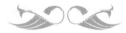

"I have read it and found it very helpful. The way it is written makes it very readable and clear and very interesting because it is written from a personal point of view."

—Southport, Merseyside (England)

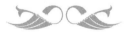

"I read your book recently, *The Do's and Don'ts of Low Blood Sugar*. I wish I had found it before I did all my technical reading. The book made me cry. It also made me feel as if I was being hugged and comforted by a dear friend. You wrote so well about all the things I've been trying to explain to my family as well as to my doctor."

—Kew Garden Hills, New York

"Roberta's personal story will not only inspire and help others, but her passion to never give up educating and creating awareness about hypoglycemia, low blood sugar, is the most inspiring of all. This book is a simple "must read" for those who never "feel right" or may have a loved one misdiagnosed for "symptoms unknown". I encourage you to support Roberta and her foundation so she can continue to make a ripple effect in the medical system and in school lunches. Hypoglycemia is real and awareness is the first line of defense for both children an adults. Keep up the great work, Roberta!"

—Sherinata Pollack

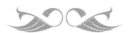

"Parker has chronic hypoglycemia; he would have symptoms daily, hospitalized frequently and struggled to stay focused in school. The Do's and Don'ts of Hypoglycemia has been a true blessing for us, Parker can relate to some of the personal stories and the information on foods, what to eliminate and what to provide has been a wonderful tool for me. The chapter of FAQ's has been a invaluable resource that we refer back to time and time again. Parker still struggles but with Roberta's book we are able to see what and where we need to change his diet to ensure he succeeds."

—Fiona Flowers

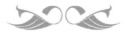

"Roberta saved my life. When I was first diagnosed I didn't know where to turn for help. I stumbled on her book at the local library and decided to contact her for some advice. I was a total stranger and this amazing angel called me weekly to give me advice and make sure I was doing okay for months. I will forever be grateful to her."

—Roseann Giannone

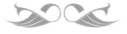

"Thank you for changing my life."

—Holland, Michigan

"I thank you once again on behalf of our patrons, and we look forward to utilizing your reference materials and to making good use of your help, and guidance in order to improve the care and services we provide to our community! May God bless you! Thanking you for your kindness."

—Dr. A. N. Malpani, M.D.
Medical Director
Bombay, India

"I am a Health Educator with the Bermuda Diabetes Association. In the last few months there has been an increase in calls from people inquiring about hypoglycemia, and nearly all of them have expressed dissatisfaction with the explanation/advice they received regarding their condition. I found your website via the Alta Vista search engine. I will recommend your book to all future callers to our Association. Thank you!"

—Jacqui Neath-Myrie
Diabetes Prevention Program Coordinator
Bermuda Diabetes Association

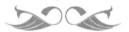

"I am a 38 year-old hypoglycemic, recently diagnosed, and I cannot thank you enough, Roberta Ruggiero. It was because of your book—*The Do's and Don'ts of Low Blood Sugar*—that I was able to recognize myself as a hypoglycemic, and I asked my doctor to test me. He, although skeptical, agreed, and to my delight my hypoglycemia was confirmed beyond a doubt. This singular diagnosis has finally explained a lifetime of symptoms, physical and emotional, and has helped me and those nearest to me understand that it was not nor is not my 'nature' to be miserable, touchy, disagreeable, negative, etc., etc., but it is only a very controllable disorder which causes me to become that way."

—Niagara Falls, New York

66 *Hi, my name is Wendy. I am a single parent of two very active daughters. For the past couple years, I would all of a sudden start to have panic attacks and thought I was going to die or maybe have a heart attack. After numerous trips to the ER, I thought I was just having panic attacks and that was it until 3 years ago, about the week before New Year's Day. I was out drinking with some friends at about 1 in the morning. I went to a local restaurant and ordered some food but didn't have a chance to eat it. I started to sweat, and friends told me I needed to go outside for some air…I never made it out the door. From what I hear, I stood up, spun around three times like a ballerina and fell through a set of glass doors and had a grand mal seizure. My friend that was with me that night is a nurse and put me on the side to prevent me from choking on my tongue. They checked my blood sugar in the ambulance and it was 24. You are supposed to be in a coma or dead if your sugar drops to 25 or below. I was very lucky. I stayed in the hospital for a week with a broken nose, a concussion and a very bad headache. I think the worst thing that happened was that when I hit the floor, I bit all the way through my tongue and almost bit half of it off. I had a hole the size of a dime in my tongue from my teeth. After that, I learned to control what I eat and hardly drink anymore. It took something like this to happen to me to make me realize that I got a second chance to live. I live every day to the fullest. I was blessed, by the glory of God, to have a friend who knew what she was doing and to the people at the hospital for quickly giving me some sugar through an IV. I hope that this story will enlighten some people on how serious hypoglycemia can be.* **Thanks.** 99

—**Wendy**

DEDICATED...

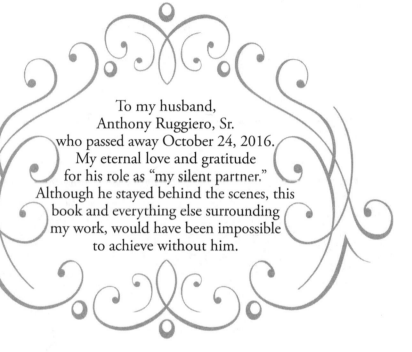

To my husband,
Anthony Ruggiero, Sr.
who passed away October 24, 2016.
My eternal love and gratitude
for his role as "my silent partner."
Although he stayed behind the scenes, this
book and everything else surrounding
my work, would have been impossible
to achieve without him.

66 *What more can I do so that my hypoglycemia doesn't turn into diabetes? I've seen the horrors and complications that it has done to my Dad and I don't want that to happen to me.* 99

—**Lisa**

TABLE OF CONTENTS

Please Note: The terms hypoglycemia and low blood sugar are used interchangeably throughout the book but have the same meaning.

ACKNOWLEDGEMENTS

The best part about writing this book is remembering everyone who played a role in its creation. They not only influenced my work, but my life.

Gratitude goes to all the people who suffer with hypoglycemia and shared their stories with me as well as every professional, medical or otherwise, who said yes to an interview. Thanks also goes to the Board of Directors, Board of Advisors, Board of Medical Advisors and all the members of The Hypoglycemia Support Foundation, Inc. (HSF), as well as the volunteers who gave so generously of their time and energy.

I would like to especially recognize the following people: Douglas M. Baird, D.O., Lorna Walker, Ph.D., Hewitt Bruce, Ph.D., Stephen J. Schoenthaler, Ph.D., Shirley S. Lorenzani, Ph.D., Nancy Appleton, Ph.D., and the late Dr. Emanuel Cheraskin, M.D., D.M.D. Each and every one of you was instrumental to my growth. As mentors, teachers, healers, and most of all friends, your direction, reassurance, and confidence gave me the courage to continue working toward my dreams.

I would like to give special thanks to Wolfram Alderson, Connie Bennett, Dr. Keith Berkowitz, Gwen Cooper, Toni Crabtree, Jan Fortgang, Valerie Goldstein, Donna Lou Guay, Annie Hart, Dr. Lynn Lafferty, Dale Ledbetter, Dr. Robert Lustig, Ken Nochimson, Tiffany Panciera, Sherinta Pollack, Carolyn Kerner Stein, Dr. Phyllis Schiffer-Simon and Leslie Lee. On a professional and personal level, each of you combined your strength and support to spur me on during my most challenging times. Whether our friendships are from the past or present, you're an inspiration to me!

Special thanks also goes to Dr. Uma Pisharody, a champion for metabolic health and nutrition, for writing the preface; to Candace Hoffmann and Melodee Putt for their valuable editing and writing suggestions. Love and deep appreciation to my niece, Lisa Piscazzi, and her son, Anthony, for sitting around the table and sharing their food, love and recipes with me. My deepest gratitude goes to Jacinta Calcut who went "above and beyond" editing this book; Don Lessne, my publisher, who still believes in me and my work after 20 years; and Elena Solis, past Graphic Designer at Frederick Fell Publishers. Each one of you gave my book extra love and tender care from the moment it was placed in your hands.

To my children, Renee and my son-in-law, Terry; Anthony and my daughter-in-law, Christina; and my late husband, Tony—your unconditional love, patience, and understanding, gave me the freedom to do my work and to make this book a reality. I am forever grateful!

To my grandchildren—Krystina, Cody, Sara, Alexa, Nicasia, Josie and Stephen and his wife Carolyn—you have made me see the world through your eyes. What more could I ask for?

Last, but definitely not least, my deepest appreciation goes to Theresa Mantovani, without whom this book would not have been possible. I miss you dearly.

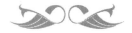

PREFACE

The Do's and Don'ts of Hypoglycemia: An Everyday Guide to Low Blood Sugar is vital for those who are looking to understand the relationship between what we eat and how we feel. It is written by a wise woman with decades of personal experience. Roberta Ruggiero was ahead of her time when she first realized the connection between excessive intake of sugar, refined carbohydrates, mood, and other symptoms of poor health. Her book not only offers help to the public looking for a resource on how to recognize symptoms of reactive or functional hypoglycemia, but also provides support, guiding them to seek out professional help and understand the importance of adhering to the required treatments.

I am a pediatric gastroenterologist often asked to consult on children with chronic symptoms, including abdominal pain, nausea, headaches, dizziness, mood swings, and fatigue. While most parents worry whether their child might have a food allergy or some type of primary gut disease, experience has taught me that many of these children feel better with lifestyle changes alone. Purely by going back to the basics of eating real food, avoiding the prepackaged, heavily processed foods and sugary drinks, which unfortunately have all too frequently become the staple diet of modern childhood, children can often find cures for their symptoms that no pill or other medication could provide.

In the last 20 years, type 2 diabetes, once thought to be an adult disease, has been affecting increasing numbers of children worldwide. Genes haven't changed; our food environment has. Our bodies, especially those of infants and toddlers, aren't made to withstand the harms from eating industrialized foods laden with sugar, additives, preservatives, and chemicals. Metabolic derangements, including impaired glucose tolerance, now affect growing numbers of children and adults, producing the symptoms that are commonly confused with other diseases.

In this edition of Roberta's book, readers should note the section discussing results of a survey conducted in conjunction with the Institute for Responsible Nutrition. Of interest, most respondents had experienced hypoglycemia after meals years before developing full-blown diabetes, highlighting an opportunity for increased awareness and preventative intervention.

More than three decades ago, long before most of today's health care professionals had even begun to recognize health risks associated with diets rich in ultra-processed foods, Roberta Ruggiero, through personal trials and tribulations, came to understand what many of us are now just starting to realize: real food is one of the most powerful medicines for both mental and physical wellbeing. Kudos to Roberta for not only transforming her own life, but for wanting to share her story with others.

—Uma Pisharody, M.D., F.A.A.P.

Seattle, Washington

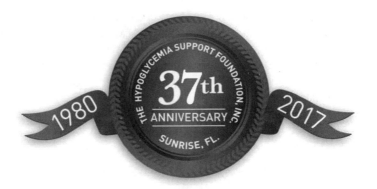

INTRODUCTION TO THE 5TH EDITION

The first edition of my book, *The Do's and Don'ts of Hypoglycemia: An Everyday Guide to Low Blood Sugar* was written in 1988. That's almost 30 years ago! And here I am, in 2017, writing the 5th Edition. It's mind boggling!

The fact that my book is still in print and going into another revision after all these years is a testament to you, my readers! You have written to me, cried on my shoulders, begged for more answers, more information and research.

From big cities such as Los Angles, California, to little-known towns such as Soddy, Tennessee; from Canada to Great Britain; from Alaska to Ireland, the letters pour in. And since The *Hypoglycemia Support Foundation, Inc.*, launched its website, www.hypoglycemia.org in 1997 and the first-ever website for *Children with Hypoglycemia* at www.hypoglycemiaKIDS.org in 2015, emails arrive on a daily basis from around the world. More often than not, I answer 400 to 500 emails a month. I correspond with hypoglycemics in China, India, Africa, Pakistan, and the Kingdom of Bahrain, right here from my office in Sunrise, Florida. How incredible God's plan!

The previous edition of my book included three areas of significant concern: hypoglycemia and children; hypoglycemia and alcoholism, and hypoglycemia and diabetes. Although I touched briefly on these topics, please realize that they all merit further attention and investigation. I also provided a special section with answers to the most commonly asked questions about hypoglycemia. There are 60 questions and answers on everything you could possibly ask or want to know about this condition. What an incredible way to learn about the highs and lows, fears and frustrations, failures and triumphs that come straight from the heart and soul of another hypoglycemic. Their questions, and how I and my medical team answered them, were too valuable and inspirational not to share. Also included in that edition was something that you were asking for, a section titled, "Smorgasbord of Dietary Delights."

And now in this 5th Edition, I am more than excited to share the results of a Hypoglycemia Questionnaire. It is a repeat of one we did in 1998. Because I combined my efforts with Wolfram Alderson, the HSF's new CEO, and Leslie Lee, our Nutritional Advisor, this newest adaptation is more medical and technical in nature and was designed to detect any possible connection between hypoglycemia and diabetes (chronically high blood glucose), particularly whether hypoglycemia is a prelude to type 2 diabetes. This was also the means used to gather information on how hypoglycemia is diagnosed, and by whom, and what kinds of treatments are beneficial, especially those related to diet. The information obtained can't be found anywhere else. Check Chapter 6 for the startling results!

Once again, it is very evident that this edition couldn't be accomplished without the teachers, advisors, and mentors who assisted me and The Hypoglycemia Support Foundation, Inc., for the past 37 years. Their time, expertise, dedication and commitment have enabled the HSF to continue to succeed, and grow beyond our wildest expectations.

I urge you now to read this book from cover to cover, especially if you or a loved one is struggling with hypoglycemia, also known as low blood sugar. It contains Gold Standard, critical information on the do's and don'ts of treating and controlling hypoglycemia symptoms through simple diet and lifestyle changes and fosters a deeper understanding of hypoglycemia—one of the most confusing, complicated, misunderstood and misdiagnosed conditions of the 21st century!

While editing this newly revised edition, one thought kept coming back to me…where would I be today if I'd had access to this information when I first got sick? Certainly, the HSF and this book wouldn't exist. I hope and pray that what I have shared in these pages will help prevent or put an end to years of suffering. It's my gift to you!

INTRODUCTION

If you think you may be going crazy; if you have thoughts of suicide; if you're constantly exhausted, anxious and depressed; if you go for weeks without a decent night's sleep; if your personality changes like the flip of a coin; if a counter full of munchies doesn't satisfy your sweet tooth; and if your doctor thinks you must be a hypochondriac because medical tests don't show anything physically wrong with you—don't despair, there's hope!

You may not need a psychiatrist, or even pain pills, tranquilizers or anti-depressants. Surprisingly, a simple DIET may relieve your symptoms!

This condition, which is confusing, complicated, misunderstood and too often misdiagnosed, is hypoglycemia, or low blood sugar. According to leading medical authorities, it affects one-half of all Americans. Books, magazines and the internet show how celebrities such as Burt Reynolds, Nicole Richie, Miley Cyrus and supermodel Carol Alt suffer from this condition. It is frightening because most people who have it don't know it. Often, the myriad collection of symptoms is blamed on other causes.

I know because I've been there. I suffered with hypoglycemia for ten years. Numerous medical specialists, dozens of tests, thousands of pills, and even the administration of electroconvulsive shock therapy (ECT) did nothing to eliminate my symptoms.

A simple glucose tolerance test (GTT), proper diet and strong determination finally led me down the road to recovery. Unfortunately, it took years. If only I had had the knowledge that lies between the covers of this book, my journey would not have been so traumatic.

To help others avoid what I experienced, to bring to them the causes and effects of hypoglycemia, and to give support, encouragement and enlightenment to those suffering from this insidious disease, I formed The Hypoglycemia Support Foundation, Inc. (HSF), on June 6, 1980.

Through the HSF, I have had the opportunity to speak with thousands of "searching" hypoglycemics. They all are looking for the best doctor, diet, book or miracle cure. They are asking the questions that I once asked: What should I eat? Should I take vitamins? Should I exercise? Why isn't my diet working? Why doesn't my family understand? Can I ever eat out again? More serious questions commonly asked are: Why doesn't my doctor recognize hypoglycemia? He says it's just a "fad" disease. Is the glucose tolerance test necessary? How can I find a physician sympathetic to a hypoglycemic's needs? The list is endless, and So sometimes, is the pain.

During this time, as I was trying to educate hypoglycemics, they, in turn, educated me. They told me what they needed and wanted and, above all, what they were not getting. I learned of their pitfalls, anxieties and fears. Echoing my own feelings, everyone I encountered seemed to respond with the same universal phrase, "If only I had known..."

There are many good books on the subject of hypoglycemia. However, whenever I insisted that a patient get a book to read about his or her condition, I began to realize that most of the people were in the first stages of hypoglycemia, a time when the mind is confused, the body is weak and concentration is difficult.

When I found myself repeating the same guidelines over and over again, I realized that these patients first needed simple, concise and comprehensible guidelines to help them handle their condition. They needed a prerequisite, a book to read BEFORE all the other books on hypoglycemia. They needed a book with specific do's and don'ts written in a layperson's vocabulary before grasping for medical definitions and explanations.

This is what I hope to achieve with *The Do's and Don'ts of Hypoglycemia*. Use it as a key to education, interweave it with commitment, and then love yourself enough to take the final step—application! Are you ready?

"To be sugar free in a sugar coated world is a nightmare!"
—**Donna 1990**

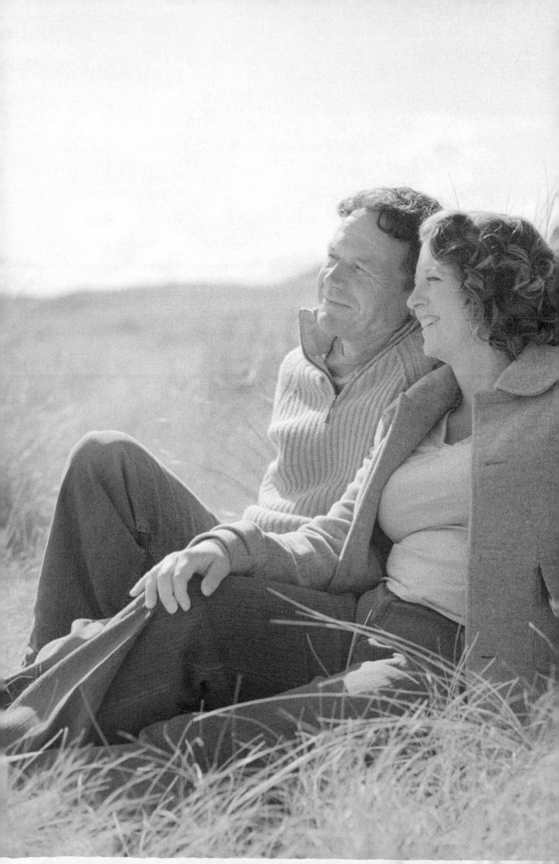

66 *I was 'diagnosed' with hypoglycemia when I was 15 years old and I am now 44. The last 5 years of my life have been sheer hell, as I have gone from doctor to doctor and always ask, "Could this have anything to do with my being hypoglycemic?" Out of over 60 doctors NOT ONE asked me about my diet and what I was doing to try and control it, so I guess I never took it seriously. It was kind of like the elephant in the room until October 10th, when I was driving home and I felt my blood sugar dropping after a full sugared up usual day, so I stopped at the store and got a large Red Bull that I took with 2 Excedrin for the headache I was developing. Long and short, I made a poor judgment call when I encountered a deer at the side of the road and chose to swerve to the other side of the road, where I miscalculated by about 6 inches, and all of a sudden my sensors on my SUV started screaming and I knew I was rolling over into the drainage ditch. I totaled my Toyota SUV and, aside from some bruises and a concussion, walked away from the accident and am now on a strict Hypo diet. Feeling pretty good today but really wondering why not one of the doctors I spoke with could have helped me with this and why nearly killing myself, thank God no one else was involved, was what it took to get me to take this diet seriously and give up my life long MAJOR addiction to sugar. Thank you for your website and the help it has given me and the encouragement I need right now.* 99

—**Deborah**

Chapter **One**
Sharing the Journey

LETTERS FROM OUR MAILBAG

Why devote a section strictly to letters and e-mails that I have received? The answer is quite simple. I am hoping the following correspondence will have the same effect on you as it had on me. I am hoping that the connection that was formed, the bond that was cemented and the feeling that flowed between the writer and me will be passed on to you, my reader. I want you to benefit by gaining inspiration from the challenges and triumphs experienced by other hypoglycemics and learn from their mistakes and their successes.

Together, let's shed more light on hypoglycemia, which it needs if the sting is to be removed from its tail. The following letters will speak for themselves.

Dear Roberta,

THANK YOU, THANK YOU, THANK YOU!

The information you have been kind enough to share with me has been the key link enabling me to return to a normal life.

Several months ago, I began growing faint and was, on about half a dozen occasions, taken to the emergency room of a local hospital. In every instance, I was told there was nothing wrong and that I was probably just hyperventilating. After consulting several doctors without any success at all, I was properly diagnosed by a local physician who recommended a glucose tolerance test. Once it was determined that I had hypoglycemia, I was referred to the Cleveland Clinic for dietary planning.

The staff at the Cleveland Clinic were enormously helpful but referred me to you and your organization for additional help. The materials you have supplied me have helped me understand my problem and do what is necessary to return to a normal life. I am saddened by my own experience with the many doctors who were unable to determine what was wrong with me. I am frightened for the many thousands of patients throughout the country with similar problems who are no doubt experiencing the same kind of difficulty with their diagnosis. I hope for their sake that they will be as fortunate as I was to be directed to you and your wonderful, caring organization.

Please let me know if there is anything I can ever do to repay the enormous debt I owe to you.

Sincerely,

Fort Lauderdale, Florida

Dear Roberta,

Thank you....Since I read your book (it saved my life, literally) about three years ago, I've been on again, and off again the diet. I usually go back on my diet after a very bad episode, such as my pancreas killing me, or I start blacking out again.

Only those who have had this devastating illness can understand how one understanding person who writes a book (you & your book) can save so many people from unnecessary reactions such as suicide.

I wrote to you once before several years ago crying my eyeballs out.

Finally, after my entire life and several doctors telling me everything but hypoglycemia, it was good to know I was not nuts.

Thank You!

Paris, Kentucky

Dear Roberta,

I have just finished reading your wonderful book for the second time, and I can't tell you how much it helped me. It's such a terrible disease to have. It was the most trying time of my whole life. I thought I was going insane for sure. It started out for me about seven months ago. I got out of bed one morning and started to have a panic attack (which I had never experienced one in my life), and thought I was having a heart attack. My husband was at work and my children, ages seven and three, were still asleep, so I called my neighbor and she took me to the hospital. They told me it was my nerves, gave me a shot and sent me home. After that I kept having panic attacks, anxiety, and severe depression. I went to my doctor and he gave me nerve pills and said that it had to be something in my subconscious that was triggering all of my symptoms. I just knew that it was something physical because I started to develop a lot of other symptoms after that. I would go back to my doctor and tell him that the pills weren't helping, about the other symptoms I was getting and he almost acted mad because I wouldn't take his word for it. I feel that God really had his hand in all of this because my family and friends were all praying for me and my neighbor (who took me to the hospital), her daughter has hypoglycemia and she thought that I could have it, because she had the same symptoms that I was having. So I went back to my doctor again and I asked him if he thought I could have low blood sugar. He sort of laughed and said that most people who have panic attacks think they have that or else a brain tumor.

I feel that he just agreed to give me a five hour GTT to humor me. I think it really offended him because I was right and he was wrong. My blood sugar level went down to 46 in the third hour of my test. When I called his office to get the results, he didn't even talk to me on the phone. His receptionist told me I had low blood sugar and made an appointment for me to see a dietitian at the hospital. She (the dietitian) was very helpful, and she even said she couldn't understand why doctors don't recognize and check people for hypoglycemia more often. Three days later I called a different doctor and made an appointment and had all of my medical records transferred over to him. Well, I am so happy that I switched doctors. My new doctor took a complete family history and said that I am a prime candidate for hypoglycemia with having diabetes in my family, and I also had diabetes with my first pregnancy. He felt that 46 on my GTT was no doubt low and he's following up on everything, too. He wants to see me every six months to check for diabetes and to see how I am doing.

I am so thankful that I didn't have to suffer a real long time, like you or some of the other poor people in your book, before I found out what was wrong. I am thankful that I now have a lot more good days than bad ones. It is so nice to have a doctor who is understanding and recognizes how dreadful it is to have this disease. I just don't understand why all doctors don't recognize hypoglycemia. It is really a shame to think that there are so many people out there who are having terrible mental and physical problems, and they probably have low blood sugar. They might never know that they can feel better just by following a diet!

Thank you for writing your book and sharing your story with so many others, I'm sure it has been very helpful to everyone who reads it, and thank you for forming the HSF.

Thank-you

Saginaw, Michigan

Dear Ms. Ruggiero,

I recently came across your book *The Do's and Don'ts of Low Blood Sugar* and would very much appreciate any information (nutritional or otherwise) you may have regarding hypoglycemia. As I began to read your book, I couldn't help but feel that I was reading my own story with all the frustrations and fears that you experienced. I would also like to say thanks for all your time and effort you put forth in getting this book published and The Hypoglycemia Foundation started.

After 10 years of being treated as a manic depressive, 20 electroconvulsive shock therapy (ECT) treatments, and being placed on every antipsychotic and antidepressant medication on the market, I was finally diagnosed as hypoglycemic. Since I have changed my diet accordingly, I feel 100% better the majority of the time.

Thank you for your time and attention you have given this letter. I have suffered quite extensively these last 15 years and have no desire to repeat this experience! Therefore, any information that you can provide me with will be most helpful.

Sincerely,

Madison, Wisconsin

Mrs. Ruggiero,

I was so happy to have found your book, *The Do's and Don'ts of Low Blood Sugar*. I'm 26 and have known for several years that I had hypoglycemia but knew little more than to stop eating sugar. I followed the "sacred diet" faithfully for years but never seemed to get much better. When I asked about what to do I was given another copy of that diet, patted on the back and was told that I would be just fine if I left the sugar alone. When I called the office confused and wilted, I was told to get a candy bar and that would bring my sugar up and I would be fine. The confusion mounted. That was when I decided I would find out on my own what I should do. So I hit the libraries, and that is where I found your book. I felt like you had written the book after spending a few months watching me. It really was nice to finally know that I was dealing with something conquerable.

Your book marks the beginning of my quest for information on this quiet culprit, who sets up camp in the corner of your life, and robs you of your senses. Even though I still find myself in unexplainable tears or wrapped in a blanket in 90 degree weather, I finally feel hope. I feel sure that God has His hand in this matter. Thank you for writing and sharing your experiences and knowledge.

God Bless You,

Milford, Michigan

Dear Mrs. Ruggiero,

I can't tell you how enlightening your book, Do's & Don'ts of Low Blood Sugar, was for me. My daughter was diagnosed with hypoglycemia in August of '91. We had been having problems with our daughter since around puberty, she is now 17. Her grades were slipping, she was always in a strange mood and her temper seemed to flash out of the blue. She just didn't seem like a happy adolescent. My daughter has always been independent and a handful but I thought these changes were just part of puberty.

When we would get on her about school she would tell us she was studying but found it hard to remember what she read. My husband and I would just shake our heads and say she just wasn't putting enough effort into her work. We even had her tested for LD problems but the test proved negative. By the time she entered high school she was having headaches, first thing in the morning, which I figured could be a migraine but she never liked school, was doing poorly, so I figured most times it was a ruse to get out of school. Then we started with dizziness and she was complaining of almost passing out. At this point we took her to the doctor. She had the Glucose Tolerance Test (over 5 hours) and was diagnosed. We were given a diet, told this was common in teens and she would probably outgrow the problem. It seemed no big deal. The doctor said to keep her on the diet for three months then start reintroducing foods looking for the dizziness as a guide. Artificial sweeteners were fine, and natural fruit juices were also acceptable, no restricted amounts.

By this time I had talked my husband into family counseling. It seemed what I thought was a family was disintegrating around me. I was an emotional mess. It never dawned on me to read up on her hypoglycemia. I could only concentrate on one thing at a time and counseling was it.

Counseling seemed to be helping out but we still had periods of uneven behavior. I had read an article in the paper about behavior problems with hypoglycemic kids and asked the doctor if this was true. He said, "No way, don't give her that handle to use." I believed him. Why? I can't answer that, not even now. After a year almost, all of the foods had been reintroduced. She has reported no dizziness but erratic behavior, even worse than before. Our counselor had her evaluated by a psychiatrist who diagnosed a long term depression. When she was arrested for battery last week I called our counselor and asked for his help. His first thought was a reevaluation. His supervisor overruled this and they had a staff meeting instead. In the meeting was the supervisor, our counselor, the psychiatrist and a psychologist. They concluded that she had a "Personality Disorder" and we had to accept her as is and we were on our own and then they wished us good luck.

Two days after this verdict my daughter brought home your book. (My daughter works at a library.) I can't even describe how I felt as I read this book. The pain, the guilt, the unbelief that I could be unaware of this for so long. That I had put my daughter through hell because I didn't do my job as a mother. I tried calling the counselor. I didn't even know if he told the staff that my daughter has hypoglycemia. We had told him when we first started the sessions. He was honest with us. He told us he knew nothing about it, we explained what we knew from the doctor and promptly forgot about it.

I don't know how to pull this together. I can't let this diagnosis stand as is if the hypoglycemia wasn't taken into account, which I feel it wasn't. I know that my daughter will not miraculously turn into Mary Poppins but if LBS accounts for even a small percentage of her problems I feel it should be reevaluated.

I need advice. I've set this trap by my own ignorance but I don't want my daughter to pay for my mistakes.

Sincerely,

Mokena, Illinois

Dear Mrs. Ruggiero,

Thank you for writing your book, *The Do's and Don'ts of Low Blood Sugar.*

In 1980 I was diagnosed as hypoglycemic by an alert and caring physician. Bless him! Even though I was not subjected to many of the horrors most hypoglycemics experience when they first realize "something" is wrong, I well remember the feeling of having been transported to some twilight zone where nothing made sense as I struggled to understand my condition. My own experience convinced me it takes two people, a knowledgeable doctor and an informed patient, to manage this condition. In my attempts to understand hypoglycemia, what it is and how to treat it, I read most of the literature available to the average person. Given my belief that education is essential to the hypoglycemic, it is still my policy to read everything available on the subject. I believe your book, *The Do's and Don'ts of Low Blood Sugar*, could be the most helpful thing a newly-diagnosed hypoglycemic could read. Its simplicity of style makes it an excellent first choice. How I wish it had been available to me in 1980.

Sincerely,

Del City, Oklahoma

I was thrilled to find Roberta Ruggiero's book, *The Do's and Don't of Low Blood Sugar*, and find out about your organization! My symptoms of hypoglycemia began in 1984 after the birth of my daughter. I knew there was nothing physically wrong with me so I thought I must have been going crazy. My mood changes were too frequent and drastic to be normal. I knew we could not afford a psychiatrist so I made an effort to cope with the problems on my own. It may have been a blessing in disguise, however, because I was not given tranquilizers and other drugs and therapy about which I've heard horror stories. My symptoms grew to include sudden hunger, weakness, dizziness, nervousness, fatigue, confusion, depression, etc. I suffered for four and a half years until finally a sympathetic doctor agreed to give me a glucose tolerance test. It was then that my suspicions were confirmed and I discovered that I was definitely hypoglycemic.

It has been almost a year since my GTT and I am finally beginning to feel that I am making progress. My doctor, sympathetic though he was, gave me the wrong advice about my diet telling me that I needed more sugar. As a result I spent about five months eating the wrong things, and my symptoms got much worse instead of better. A friend recognized what was happening to me and put me on the right track. I am doing much better now, but am still not as well as I would like to be.

That is the reason I was so glad to find Mrs. Ruggiero's book. I was beginning to lose ground and get depressed about my condition again, feeling that it was a never-ending battle. The book was a tremendous lift to my spirits and renewed my courage to keep up the pace on the road to recovery. I wish that every person who has hypoglycemia or is suffering the symptoms and doesn't know the cause could read this book. It is a great support!

Thank you so much for such a helpful book and for letting me share my story with you, though I'm sure you've heard it hundreds of times from others! Thank you for all you are doing to help others with hypoglycemia!

Yours truly,

Selma, North Carolina

Dear Mrs. Ruggiero,

I read your book recently *The Do's and Don'ts of Low Blood Sugar*. I wish I had found it before I did all my technical reading. The book made me cry. It also made me feel as if I was being hugged and comforted by a dear friend. You wrote so well about all the things I've been trying to explain to my family, as well as to my doctor.

Sincerely,

Kew Garden Hills, New York

Dear Roberta,

Thank you so much for your call. I can't tell you how honored I felt. Since I got over the shock that my condition was "nutritional" and not "mental," I always felt that there was something I should be doing so that others would not needlessly have to go through what I went through. You took that step and I hope that I can contribute to help spread the word!

Sincerely,

Topeka, Kansas

Dear Dr. Ruggiero,

My name is Kate and I am a hypoglycemic. I would like to share my story. I am 18 years old, and I was recently diagnosed with the condition about three months ago. Up until then, the doctors didn't know what was wrong with me. When I was 14, I suffered three concussions (from soccer) and ever since then I've had a non-stop headache. They wrote it off as a post concussive syndrome, but little did they know that it was really all from my low blood sugar. I've had a non-stop headache since November 2, 1997. I had other symptoms that related to the symptoms of hypoglycemia. The doctors put me on every medication you can think of, ranging from anti-depressants to anti-seizure medication. I never saw any change, nothing made the pain stop, only certain things made it worse (stress). Throughout the whole four years I was never depressed though, it was strictly for the use of stopping the headache, which it never did. Hypoglycemia is in my family, but I never knew I had it, until I gave up soda for Lent this year, 2002, and when I had a small little piece of candy, my headache tripled. So then I asked my doctor what was wrong and he had no clue, he said I might have an allergy to sugar, and so I asked him how we find out, and then I proceeded with the five-hour glucose testing. It was a real shock when the tests came back positive for hypoglycemia. If I didn't stop the soda, I never would have figured it out.

The doctors always threw medicine at me and never once thought to check my blood. From that day on I started seeing a nutritionist and my health has dramatically changed. For the first time in four and a half years I actually felt like I had hope and that I knew I was going to get better. I've been on an amino acid drink, which has helped me so much, and I'm currently trying to get off my medication. I've seen such a difference, that I wish the doctors would have figured it out back then."

Sincerely,

Kate

"Please don't tell me I can never, ever eat a hot fudge sundae!"
—**Helena 2001**

MY PERSONAL EXPERIENCES

There was no turning back. After years of trying to hide my deepest secret, I was now sharing it with what seemed to be the world. Tallahassee's *Capitol News* quoted me verbatim on May 9, 1978: It stated that Roberta Ruggiero, a former shock treatment patient from Cooper City, called the therapy "barbaric" saying she would "rather die than go through electric shock again."

The trail from private mental patient to public notoriety started out rather innocently. After my first child was born in 1961, I went into a deep depression. I couldn't stop crying. I had heard of postpartum depression, but mine was a deluge of tears that had no end. My family physician kept assuring me that my reaction was normal and that it would go away. When it didn't, he introduced me to my first tranquilizer—Valium.

Then the headaches started. The pain was there in the morning when I woke up and persisted through my waking hours and sometimes through the night. The pounding got so intense it felt as though my heart was actually throbbing inside my head. I was then given pills to reduce the pain.

I began having difficulty sleeping at night. Trying to get up in the morning was even more of a task. I became tired and weak. Cooking and cleaning the house, which I had always enjoyed, became a dreaded chore. I began to skip breakfast, hardly ate lunch and just nibbled at dinner...if I had the energy to cook.

In 1963, I gave birth to my second child. All of my previous symptoms were compounded by dizzy spells and blurred vision. My nerves, needless to say, were hopelessly frazzled. My hands and feet were constantly cold to the point of feeling frostbitten. Even with medication, my symptoms got progressively worse. My doctor put me in the hospital for a multitude of tests: laboratory, x-rays, spinal taps and electroencephalogram. All the tests came out negative. There was nothing physically wrong with me. I began to think, beyond a doubt, that I was going crazy. I withdrew into a shell, avoiding contact with my family and friends because I was too embarrassed and ashamed to face them.

It was at this point that my doctor recommended psychotherapy. I spent several months with the first psychiatrist. He thought that perhaps the strain of getting married at an early age (18) and having two children 16 months apart were the major contributing factors to my illness.

Maybe a "contributing factor," but not THE reason. When the psychiatrist put me on heavy doses of anti-depressants, I went to psychiatrist number two. It was a repeat performance.

My pain and symptoms were being drowned with strong medication. I was given pills to calm me down, pills to help me sleep and pills to relieve pain. That was the order of the day. But since medication and therapy were not enough to relieve the symptoms, much less stabilize them, a third psychiatrist suggested electroconvulsive shock therapy (ECT), known simply as shock treatments! By this time, I was desperate and would have tried anything. The year was 1969, and in addition to all of my physical and emotional pain, I began to feel guilty about what I was putting my husband through. I agreed to go away and have what I believed was the "cure"—my last hope.

I was wrong. I had not anticipated that my hospital room would have bars on the windows and doors. I didn't know that my clothing, wedding ring and "Miraculous Medal" would be taken away. And even more frightening were the screams, stares and glassy eyes of the patients who had already received treatments. I'll never forget the cot and its leather straps that bound my hands and feet, the electrodes that were put on my temples, and the rubber gag inserted in my mouth. The memories haunt me to this day.

After my first treatment, while I still had some faculties intact, I begged to go home, or at least speak to my husband. If he knew what I was going through, he would stop them. They said no. I had signed the papers for a series of electric shock treatments, and that's what I was going to get.

I had eight treatments in eleven days. The results were horrifying. I am thankful I don't remember all of them. I do remember feeling like I was in a state of limbo. My mind was functioning, but not in coordination with the rest of my body. Despair, shame, guilt and thoughts of suicide remained. Approximately ten months later, I reluctantly agreed to another series of treatments but, this time, on an outpatient basis. It was at the end of this series that I swore I would rather die than ever be subjected to electric shock treatments again. The physical pain was nothing compared to the feelings of isolation, embarrassment and humiliation.

With no solution in sight, we took the advice of our family physician, who suggested that a change of scenery or a move to another state might offer some relief. It would be like a fresh start. Therefore, when my husband had an opportunity to move to South Florida, we didn't hesitate.

Our move was exciting. I began to feel a little better. The pain in my head began to go away. Just having the sun shine every day seemed to promise a future where none had existed for so long. Then, suddenly, it happened again. This time, though, a new symptom assailed me. I began having fainting spells. I agreed to go for one last medical consultation. Dr. Arthur Ecoff, an osteopathic physician, examined me, reviewed my records and suggested a glucose tolerance test. I had never had this test before and was skeptical that a diagnosis could be reached. At this point, I would have settled for any diagnosis!

The GTT was taken and I was told I had a severe case of functional hypoglycemia. I was ecstatic! At last, I had a diagnosis, a name and a cure! But, to both my bewilderment and surprise, instead of a bottle of pills, injections or vitamins, I was given a DIET! Goodbye Yankee Doodles, Devil Dogs, hot fudge sundaes and apple pie. Hello chicken, fish, fresh vegetables, whole grains and fruits. I thought, "This is going to be a cinch."

Unfortunately, what I hoped would be an "overnight" remedy turned out to take several years of sorting through a mass of confusing and complicated information. Due to the unfamiliarity with the stages of recuperation, the controversy surrounding its treatment, and non-acceptance from many in the medical community, I found myself with the feeling of being the only person in the world suffering from this baffling disease.

Eventually, success did come, but alleviating my symptoms was a long and slow process. It would have been quicker if only I had understood the importance of individualizing my diet, the necessity for vitamins and exercise, and the role a positive attitude plays in the healing process. Above all, if there were other hypoglycemics to lend support and encouragement, the road back to health would not have been so rocky. Faith, patience, determination and the boundless love of my family were the cornerstones to my recovery.

Consequently, I didn't hesitate for a moment when I came across an article in *The Miami Herald* appealing to anyone who had experienced the devastating effects of electric shock treatments. A committee for patients' rights was lobbying in Tallahassee and, after listening to my story, was eager to have me testify before the state legislature on behalf of mental patients. My hope was to convince the lawmakers to put severe restrictions on the use of ECT and, better yet, give the glucose tolerance test before its administration.

Little did I know that my life would never be the same. My story appeared in newspapers and on radio stations. I was immediately inundated with phone calls and mail from all over the state.

Letters like the following became all too familiar.

> "Please send information. I had undiagnosed hypoglycemia for 23 years, and during that time, I ran the whole gamut—depression, weight gain, weight loss, anxiety, psychiatric therapy and institutionalization—until the proper diagnosis was reached. The glucose tolerance test revealed that I had a blood sugar level of 35! Since that time, I am like a new person. I follow the proper diet, enjoy life and have no apprehension about blacking out without notice."

> "I was ecstatic to see your article. My case was diagnosed approximately four months ago by my chiropractor. My internist had written me off as either psychotic or a hypochondriac, or both."

This feedback was the inspiration for my decision to start speaking to both hypoglycemics and members of our community.

When I couldn't handle the flood of letters and phone calls, and when I realized I needed medical and professional guidance, the idea to form a support group became a reality.

So the formation of The Hypoglycemia Research Foundation, Inc., became official on June 6, 1980. The organization was renamed The Hypoglycemia Support Foundation, Inc., on December 13, 1991. I am proud to say that I believe that no other organization has accomplished so much with so little.

When I say "little," I refer to practically no money, secretarial services, office equipment, supplies, private phone or office space. How did we survive? Through positive people, positive thoughts, endless hours of hard work, dedication and prayer—plenty of prayer.

For seventeen years, from 1980 to 1997, the HSF held monthly meetings. We had medical or professional speakers share their knowledge of hypoglycemia, whether it was from a medical, nutritional, psychological or holistic point of view. We participated in health fairs and seminars while I personally brought the message about hypoglycemia to local organizations, schools and hospitals.

In 1984, I was proud and honored to be coordinator of a research project studying the correlation between diet and behavior in juvenile delinquents. It was under the direction of Stephen J. Schoenthaler, Ph.D., a professor of criminal justice at California State University, Stanislaus. With the help and guidance of Dr. Douglas M. Baird, Dr. Lorna Walker, and Nutritional Biochemist, Jay Foster, the study was conducted at The Starting Place in Hollywood, Florida. The participants were 35 juvenile delinquents willing to find out if there might be a nutritional and physical cause to their behavior.

We tested them physically, psychologically, nutritionally, and chemically. The results, though not conclusive due to lack of a placebo control group, are published in the book *Nutrition and Brain Function* (Craiger Press, Basle, Switzerland, 1987) Future studies using control groups and other scientific criteria are absolutely necessary in this area.

In 1988, I wrote the first edition of *The Do's and Don'ts of Low Blood Sugar: An Everyday Guide to Hypoglycemia.* It was the core of all that I had learned since finally being diagnosed. I wanted to share it in the hope of sparing other hypoglycemics the pain and suffering I went through.

In 1993, a revised edition of my book came out with two additional chapters. "Letters From Our Mailbag" was a hit with our readers. Hypoglycemics, sharing their experiences, convinced my readers that they were not alone and there was indeed help at hand.

For the next five years, I kept a low profile with the HSF. I needed time to find out exactly what role my organization should play and what course of action I must take. During this time of reassessment, I took a leap of faith and launched the HSF's first website, www.hypoglycemia.org. What a journey it has been. I've seen our visitor numbers climb to almost 1,000,000 as of this writing. Over 5500 have responded to our hypoglycemia/diabetes survey, and e-mails and requests for information have come in from 25 countries!

Take a look at what we have accomplished, past and present!

• Publication of an award-winning book on hypoglycemia with praise from the American Library Association – 5th edition available in 2017.

• Designed and distributed a wide range of educational materials, including brochures titled "Hypoglycemia & Children: Is Your Child At Risk?" and "Hypoglycemia & Alcoholism: The Missing Link to Recovery."

• Provided hundreds of educational presentations, support meetings, health fairs, and lectures at schools, hospitals and businesses.

- Served as champion for over a million patients with misdiagnosed metabolic conditions (e.g., hypoglycemia) - and responded to over 100,000 inquiries and emails from every state in the U.S. and countries around the world.

- Garnered extensive earned media and maintained an informative presence on social media.

- Built a global following and community via the www.hypoglycemia.org website.

- Serving as a pediatric advocate, established the only website dedicated to children suffering from hypoglycemia: www.hypoglycemiaKIDS.org.

- Shared inspiration and expertise with the international movement addressing hypoglycemia.

- Now, this book is in its fifth printing with a revised edition. It was written with the same hope of sparking your enthusiasm and planting the seeds of determination, strength and persistence. You need it all in order to learn every single thing about controlling hypoglycemia before it controls you!

I have cried three times today. But reading the stories in your book has helped me so much!
—**Vanessa January 2008**

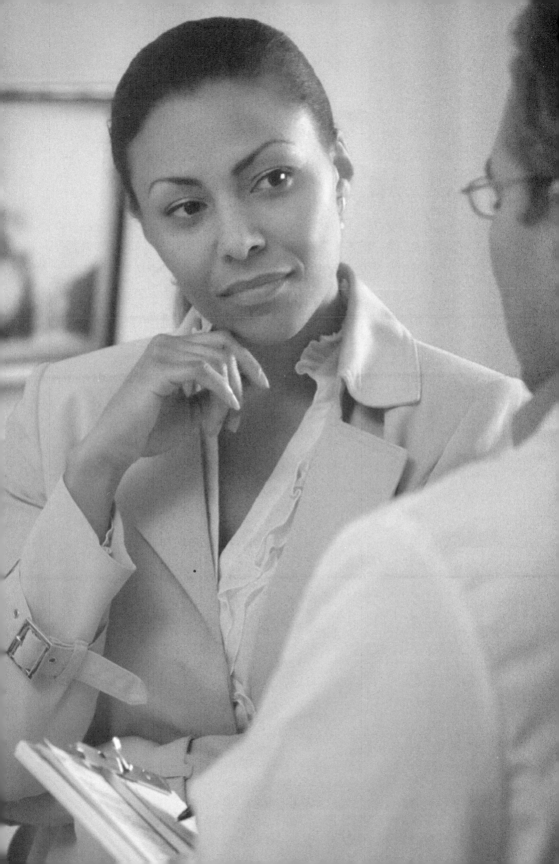

66 *I am so relieved. My doc gave me only a list of suggested mini-meals as a means of dealing with my new diagnosis. Your suggestion of my keeping a log, recording foods (and when) I eat and my responses is great. It hadn't occurred to me to do that. Now I realize why, perhaps, I have hand tremors, blurred vision, am very emotional, find it hard to concentrate, am indecisive, etc. Thank you!* 99

— Nan
June 2007

Chapter Two
Getting started

DEFINITION OF HYPOGLYCEMIA

I've read and reread the definition of hypoglycemia at least a hundred times. I've been asked repeatedly, "What is hypoglycemia?" And, in turn, I have asked the leading authorities in the fields of preventive and nutritional medicine. Their answers, although similar, are varied. Some are more technical than others. One thing is for certain—the definition of hypoglycemia can be as diversified and complex as the condition itself, or as simple and easy as some of the steps to control it.

In simple layman's language, hypoglycemia is the body's inability to properly handle the large amounts of sugar that the average American consumes today. It's an overload of sugar, alcohol, caffeine, tobacco and stress.

In medical terms, hypoglycemia is defined in relation to its cause. Functional hypoglycemia, the kind we are addressing here, is the over secretion of insulin by the pancreas in response to a rapid rise in blood sugar or "glucose."

All carbohydrates (vegetables, fruits and grains, as well as simple table sugar) are broken down into simple sugars by the process of digestion. This sugar enters the bloodstream as glucose, and our level of blood sugar rises. The pancreas then secretes a hormone known as insulin into the blood in order to bring the glucose down to normal levels.

In hypoglycemia, the pancreas sends out too much insulin and the blood sugar plummets below the level necessary to maintain wellbeing.

Since all the cells of the body, especially the brain cells, use glucose for fuel, a blood glucose level that is too low starves the cells of needed fuel, causing both physical and emotional symptoms.

Some of the symptoms of hypoglycemia are:

Fatigue, insomnia, mental confusion, nervousness, mood swings, faintness, headaches, depression, phobias, heart palpitations, craving for sweets, cold hands and feet, forgetfulness, dizziness, blurred vision, inner trembling, outbursts of temper, sudden hunger, allergies and crying spells.

After reading a list like this, one can see why hypoglycemia could be misunderstood and easily misdiagnosed. Don't be alarmed if you read other books that I recommend and see that the list is, in fact, even longer. Don't be confused and frightened when you read other definitions that range from a paragraph to several pages in length.

For the beginner, it is important that you first recognize that most often hypoglycemia is the result of a diet high in sugar, alcohol, caffeine and tobacco.

Before going any further, look at your dietary habits and/or any addictive traits. Start adding up the sodas, coffee, cakes and cigarettes you consume in one day. Keep track of how many meals you miss. Are you under a tremendous amount of stress with your spouse, children, boss, etc.? All of these circumstances can give birth to a case of low blood sugar that can plague you for the rest of your life. Don't take your body for granted. Neglect it, and you'll pay a high price. Take care of it, and low blood sugar becomes an inconvenience that you can manage by yourself.

IS THERE A DOCTOR OUT THERE?

The phone rang and I didn't want to answer it. I was going to be late for an appointment 20 minutes away. Reluctantly, I picked up the receiver, and a woman's voice said, "Is this The Hypoglycemia Support Foundation?"

"Yes. May I help you?" I asked. She proceeded to tell me her story. It was one that I had heard hundreds of times before, but the tone of her voice was more despondent.

Usually, I can listen attentively, but this time my mind was on my appointment. "Please give me your name and address, and I'll send you some literature."

But the frail voice continued to speak. "Please, please help me. I'm begging you—find me a doctor immediately. I'm anxious and depressed. I can't sleep at night, and I can't get up in the morning. I have an incredible craving for sweets. I read an article on hypoglycemia and believe that could be my problem. When I asked my present physician to give me a glucose tolerance test, he refused. He prescribed Valium. Please, before I get hooked on tranquilizers, I want to see a doctor who will listen to me."

I shuddered, and my heart sank. An overwhelming feeling of helplessness set in. I forgot about my appointment and listened to the tortured voice of a person in distress. I wondered to myself, as I had many times before, how many more stories like this one will I have to hear? When will hypoglycemia be accepted as a genuine and serious illness? My own experience and the experience of thousands of others demonstrate that hypoglycemia is real. It does exist. When will the medical profession take it seriously?

In 1980, when I formed the HSF, I wrote to about 50 local physicians looking for help and guidance. I was desperately seeking to arrange places to send the numerous patients who kept asking me where to go for treatment. No one responded. Discouraged and disillusioned, I decided to move beyond my local sphere of influence and contact physicians around the country who knew about hypoglycemia. Astonishingly, a number of them answered.

Emanuel Cheraskin, M.D., D.M.D., Harvey M. Ross, M.D., Jeffrey Bland, Ph.D., E. Marshall Goldberg, M.D., Carlton Fredericks, Ph.D., and Robert S. Mendelsohn, M.D., all responded, offering encouragement, support, guidance and hope. Although I was optimistic that I would hear from them, I think— deep down inside—I was surprised. Probably because I knew the recent history of hypoglycemia. In the late 1960s and early 1970s, hypoglycemia was written up in a large number of lay publications. The disease suddenly became trendy. It was used as a way to explain some of the worst ills of humanity with little or no scientific backing, and a number of people proclaimed themselves to be hypoglycemics without bothering to consult a doctor or get a glucose tolerance test. The backlash in the medical establishment was swift. In 1949, the American Medical Association (AMA) awarded Dr. Seale Harris its highest honor for the research that led to the discovery of hypoglycemia. After the flood of quackery and self-diagnosis began, the AMA, in 1973, did a 180-degree turn and labeled hypoglycemia a "non-disease."

Don't let this discourage you. There are doctors out there. As the HSF started to gain recognition, acceptance and credibility, doctors from all fields of medicine volunteered their services. From general practitioners in the medical field to osteopaths, chiropractors, nutritionists, and dietitians, they all came. They lectured at our meetings, held seminars, wrote articles and served on our board of directors.

Don't give up so easily. Take your time, have a positive attitude and follow the HSF's simple guidelines in your search for that special "healer."

THE DO's OF HYPOGLYCEMIA

DO HAVE someone go with you on your first visit. Sometimes, the first visit is an emotional one, and you may be nervous or apprehensive. Consequently, questions and/or answers may be misinterpreted or misunderstood. Having a second party along usually helps.

DO BRING a written list of symptoms, past medical records and personal recollections relating to your present problems. The importance of your past history and the sequence of events leading up to your present condition cannot be overemphasized.

DO BRING in a diet/symptom diary. It should include a list of everything you have eaten, including any medication you may have taken, in the previous five to seven days. Try to list the time eaten and any symptoms or reactions following consumption. This is important and can be a useful tool for the physician in diagnosing hypoglycemia. However, if you are physically and emotionally unable to do it, DO NOT PANIC—a diagnosis can still be made without it. Bring in your list of questions. Ask them one at a time, and make sure you understand the answer before going on to the next.

DO TELL the physician about any medication you may be taking at the time. Certain medications cannot be tolerated by hypoglycemics.

DO WRITE down instruction or record them, whatever is easier for you.

DO DISCUSS in detail your feelings or concerns, not just your symptoms. If you have fears you are not expressing, your treatment will be longer, more difficult and far more expensive.

DO BE specific and to the point. The more prepared you are, the better equipped the doctor will be to make a proper diagnosis.

DO FIND out if your physician is associated with a hospital in case of an emergency.

DO DISCUSS costs and insurance information. Insurance companies differ on their policies and willingness to pay for various tests and procedures. Is your doctor willing to work out a payment arrangement and/or accept whatever the insurance company pays?

DO GET a second opinion, especially if you are not completely satisfied with the first physician.

DO CHECK the office procedures and staff. Do they overbook? Are they friendly? Are they helpful? The last thing you need is a doctor too busy to listen or who makes you feel uncomfortable.

DO CHOOSE a competent, caring, and trustworthy physician who respects your individuality. The doctor-patient relationship is crucial. If your doctor doesn't have your complete confidence or isn't meeting your special needs, then it's definitely time to change.

DO NOTIFY the physician's office, preferably in writing, if you are upset with the conduct or services of either the physician or the staff.

DO DISCUSS a complete prevention program. You need to know how to avoid future health problems, not just how to eliminate the ones you have now. Your current problems are not the only issues that need to be addressed.

DO BE leery of alternative or new treatments that promise or claim to be a cure-all.

DO CARRY a Health Emergency Card if you're experiencing many LBS symptoms, especially if you've recently blacked-out or fainted. You can keep your card in your purse, car or briefcase—any place that can be seen in case of emergency.

THE DON'Ts OF HYPOGLYCEMIA

DON'T CALL your physician DEMANDING a glucose tolerance test after listening to the news or reading an article on hypoglycemia. Instead, write down this information as well as a list of your symptoms and the reasons why you feel the test is necessary. Make an appointment to see your physician, and present him with all the information. If he appears inattentive or cannot give you a seemingly justifiable reason why you should not have the test, look for another physician.

DON'T STAY with a physician you cannot communicate with or feel confident about. It will only complicate existing problems.

DON'T CALL your physician unnecessarily. If your questions can wait, write them down and save them for the next visit. The physician will likely have more time then to give you a better explanation.

DON'T WAIT to call your physician if you're in pain, your symptoms are persistent, or last several days.

DON'T CONTINUE to be a patient of any physician who just listens for a few minutes and says your symptoms are "all in your head." If you are given a prescription for Valium, get a second opinion as soon as possible.

DON'T WITHHOLD any medical history out of fear or embarrassment. It is necessary for a proper diagnosis.

DON'T SEEK the advice of a physician and then not follow the instructions issued to you. It's a waste of time and money.

DON'T RUN from one doctor to another. Give each one at least two to four visits to help you.

DON'T AVOID going to a physician. If your symptoms persist after you've put yourself on a hypoglycemic diet, seek medical advice.

DON'T AVOID a physician because you lack insurance or money. Ask a family member or friend for financial assistance. You can't afford not to.

If it is hypoglycemia, the faster you are diagnosed and treated, the sooner you'll recover.

DON'T DEMAND to be unnecessarily hospitalized.

DON'T HESITATE to speak up—ask questions. If you're too timid or embarrassed to communicate with your doctor, then he/she won't be able to adequately meet your needs.

DON'T COMPARE your program or progress with someone else's. Each person's emotional, physical and spiritual make-up is unique. A competent physician will tailor a program to fit your individual needs.

DON'T FORGET, there ARE many caring, sensitive, trustworthy physicians out there. If at first you don't succeed in finding one—try, try again!

DON'T RELY solely on an internet recommendation or review of a physician. Try to speak directly with someone who has been to that doctor or who knows a satisfied patient.

Nothing takes the place of a personal recommendation.

DON'T ORDER medication on the internet thinking it will solve your hypoglycemia problems. For reactive/functional hypoglycemia, DIET is the cornerstone treatment!

DON'T JUMP into anything online that promises, "This will cure your hypoglycemia." Proceed with caution. Do not rush to take their suggestions or to buy their recommended products. Compare and be informed from reliable sources.

"There are 39 people in my family with sugar problems. Some have diabetes, some hypoglycemia. It will be a blessing to get help."
—Ramona 2002

" *I first met Roberta in Miami and saw first-hand the helpful way in which she was trying to spread the word and offer information for those who might have hypoglycemia. I was very moved that she would spend selfless hours each day writing or calling others who needed help and who seemed not to have any idea what might be wrong with them. Roberta offered hope and possible answers.*

Coincidentally, it was at the same time that close members of my own family realized that they too had hypoglycemia. Their ages ranged from sixteen to forty. Each symptom was different but debilitating for my cousins. The forty year old would feel faint and extremely grouchy. One of the teenagers became very angry when he had not eaten and the other had symptoms of depression. Her sleep was affected and her eating was erratic, actually I should say—not eating.

The family took them to doctor after doctor with little results. Finally the older cousin had a diagnosis. As soon as he got control of his diet —for him, with protein and nuts, his mood swings left. He also was advised to reduce his sugar intake. Once the sixteen year old boy was told that diet was affecting his life, he was put on an eating regimen. He too needed protein. As an athlete, by altering his eating habits, his athletics improved and his anger disappeared if he ate his meals. The female teenager had more difficulty at first since her symptoms were more severe. Again, once she started to acknowledge that what she was putting in her mouth directly affected her mood, her symptoms started to dissipate. Helpful answers were right in front of them—food.

They were all given a copy of Roberta's book, The Do's and Don'ts of Hypoglycemia, and this became daily reading. Since hypoglycemia appears to be in my family, I have become very aware of food choices as well.

The remarkable changes in life as a result of Roberta's dedication are very inspiring. Some of the stories break your heart—that people had to suffer so long when help was so close by—in some cases—in their own refrigerator.

This work and book are important! "

—Barrie Brett
Author/Award-Winning Producer

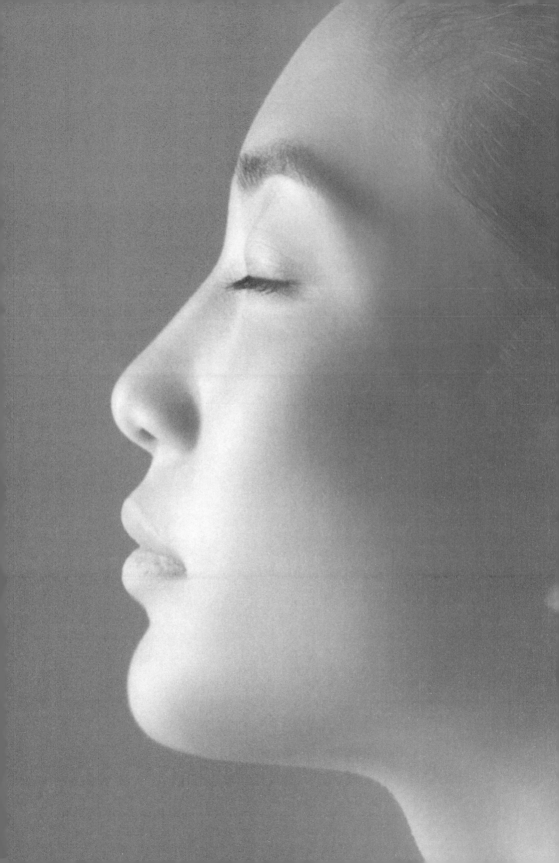

66 Thank you for your book, and thank you for your efforts! Your book made me feel less... helpless. I also wanted to let you know that since I have been attempting to manage my symptoms, I have been seeing my old self return. I welcome him back, so does my wife.99

—**Brock**

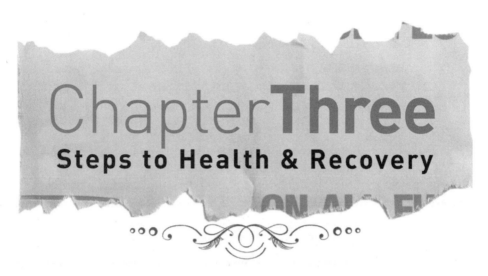

ChapterThree
Steps to Health & Recovery

THE IMPORTANCE OF INDIVIDUALIZING YOUR DIET

One of the HSF members called to tell me she was feeling terrible, particularly after eating breakfast. She started to shake, her stomach was nauseous and she felt jittery throughout the morning. She didn't understand why her symptoms were getting worse even though she was staying on a strict diet—no sugar, white flour, caffeine, alcohol or tobacco.

I suggested that we go over her diet, but she emphatically said, "It can't be my diet. I eat only what my doctor told me to eat and what the books I read suggested." However, upon my insistence, she started to give me an account of her daily intake of food. First thing every morning, she drank an eight-ounce glass of orange juice. Even though the book she read said to take four ounces, she figured eight should be twice as good.

I didn't let her continue any further. From my own personal experiences, there is no way I can handle orange juice on an empty stomach first thing in the morning. A 12-ounce glass of orange juice, although it is "natural," contains nine teaspoons of sugar. For me and many hypoglycemics that I have spoken to, orange juice causes the same reaction as a strong cup of black coffee. The results are the shakes, butterflies in the stomach and an overall feeling of wanting to "jump out of your skin."

At first, it was difficult for this hypoglycemic to understand that if she had this "nervous attack" every morning after eating the same breakfast, she should begin to question her diet—not continue to abide by it when she suffered adverse symptoms. We are individuals and thus must tailor every diet to our own bodies when a given diet proves troublesome.

As I mentioned before, there are many books on hypoglycemia. If you've read some of them, by now you're aware that many disagree on what type of diet to follow. It's indeed confusing if you read one book and it tells you to eat a high protein/low carbohydrate diet, while another book says to consume low protein/high carbohydrate foods. Where does that leave you, the confused and bewildered hypoglycemic?

First of all, I am sure that each author has enough confirmation and evidence that his or her diet is successful. Most likely, they all are. Probably, this is due to the fact that the big offenders (sugar, white flour, alcohol, caffeine and tobacco) are eliminated and six small meals are consumed instead.

But the key to a successful diet lies in its "individualization." Each one of us is different. Each one of us is biochemically unique. Therefore, every diet must be tailor-made to meet our individual nutritional requirements.

The list of foods your physician gives you or the list you may read in your favorite book on hypoglycemia, even the suggested foods list in the back of this book, are basic guidelines. Variations come with time and patience, trial and error. Don't be afraid to listen to your body. It will send you signals when it cannot tolerate a food.

So basically stick to the suggestions in the following do's and don'ts, and hopefully, with just a few adjustments during your course of treatment, a new and healthier you will gradually appear.

THE DO's OF HYPOGLYCEMIA

DO KEEP a daily account of everything you eat for one week to ten days. In one column, list every bit of food, drink and medication that you take and at what time. In the second column, list your symptoms and the time at which you experience them. Very often you will see a correlation between what you have consumed and your symptoms. When you do, eliminate those foods or drinks that you notice are contributing to your behavior and note the difference. DO NOT STOP MEDICATION. If you believe that your medication may be contributing to your symptoms, contact your physician. A diet diary is your personal blueprint—a clear overall view of what you are eating, digesting and assimilating. It can be the first indicator that something is wrong and, perhaps, a very inexpensive way of correcting a very simple problem.

DO START eliminating the "biggies"—those foods, drinks and chemicals that cause the most problems: sugar, white flour, alcohol, caffeine and tobacco.

DO BE extremely careful when and how you eliminate the offending substances. Only YOU, with the guidance of a healthcare professional, can decide. Some patients chose to go at a steady pace. If you drink 4-6 cups of coffee a day, gradually reduce consumption over a period of days or weeks. The same is true for food or tobacco. If you are heavily addicted to all of the aforementioned, particularly alcohol, then withdrawal should not be attempted unless you are under the care of a physician.

DO REPLACE offending foods immediately with good, wholesome, nutritious food and snacks as close to their natural state as possible. Lean meats, poultry (without the skin), whole grains, vegetables and allowable fruits are recommended. We want to prevent deprivation from setting in, especially the "poor me, I have nothing to eat" attitude. There is plenty to eat.

DO EAT six small meals a day or three meals with snacks in between. Remember not to overeat.

DO DRINK plenty of water. Most physicians say eight glasses of water a day is best.

DO BE aware that when you start on a hypoglycemic diet, you might experience migrating aches, pain in your muscles and/or joints, headaches or extreme fatigue. This is normal when eliminating refined foods. Call your physician if they persist.

DO BE prepared to keep your blood sugar stabilized at all times, whether at home, the office, at school or traveling. At home you should always have allowable foods ready in the refrigerator or cupboards. Always keep snacks in your car or where you work.

DO PACKAGE food in Tupperware or air-tight containers. Aladdin's insulated thermos jar is handy for cold food and snacks. Aladdin also sells wide-mouth, insulated bottles for hot foods, like soups or cut up meat and vegetables. Packaged nuts, seeds, and cheese can be easily carried or stored in a purse or in jacket pockets. You can buy almost everything you need at a supermarket.

DO ROTATE your foods. Eating the same foods over and over again for consecutive days can result in food sensitivities or allergies.

DO READ labels. Avoid ALL sugars—dextrose, fructose, glucose, lactose, maltose and sucrose. Read labels in health food stores too. Just because you buy something in a health food store does not necessarily mean you can tolerate the ingredients.

DO AVOID artificial sweeteners, additives, preservatives and food coloring. Monosodium Glutamate (MSG) is a big problem for many hypoglycemic. Avoid it completely.

DO WATCH your fruit consumption. If you are in the early or severe stages of hypoglycemia, you may not be able to eat any fruit. Some patients can eat just a small amount. Your diet diary will help guide you. Avoid dried fruits completely.

DO BE careful of the amount of "natural" foods or drinks you consume. Even though juices are natural, they contain high amounts of sugar. Whether or not the sugar you consume is natural, your body doesn't know the difference. Sugar is sugar, and your body will react to an excess of it.

DO DILUTE your juices, using about 2/3 juice to 1/3 water. If that's still too strong for you, try 1/2 juice and 1/2 water. Drink small quantities or drink them after you have eaten something, especially if you find that taking them on an empty stomach causes you problems.

DO BE inventive. Introduce new, unprocessed foods that have no preservatives, additives or chemicals. Look especially for whole grains and vegetables.

DO ARRANGE food to look palatable.

DO BROIL, bake or steam food.

DO ATTEND some natural cooking classes. You will be taught to reduce sugar, salt, saturated fats, cholesterol and allergenic foods from your diet and still enjoy eating. Call your local schools, libraries and health food stores, or scan the local papers to find out what is available in your area.

DO UNDERSTAND the meaning of "enriched." It does not mean extra amounts of vitamins. It means a small amount of some of the vitamins that were processed out of the food has been replaced.

DO HAVE your family stick to some of the basic principles of your diet. The big NO's for a hypoglycemic (sugar, white flour, alcohol, tobacco and caffeine) are detrimental to anyone's health.

DO CHANGE your attitude about what constitutes a snack. We tend to think of snacks in terms of goodies or sweet treats. A good snack can be a half-baked sweet potato with broccoli, half-stuffed tomato with tuna fish, some steamed zucchini and onions on a half cup of brown rice, a chicken leg or a slice of turkey.

DO SERIOUSLY consider going to OA (Overeaters Anonymous) or AA (Alcoholics Anonymous). Many HSF members found these meetings to be very helpful in controlling their addictions to sugar and food in general.

DO BE aware of the fact that some medications contain caffeine. If you're having reactions to the following medications, bring this matter to the attention of your physician: Anacin, APC, Caffergot, Coricidin, Excedrin, Fiorinal, Four-Way Cold Tablets and Darvon Compound, etc.

DO WEIGH yourself every day. Be aware of weight gain and weight loss. This is vital information in maintaining good health.

DO CHECK into other areas if you don't make progress with dietary changes. Hypoglycemia has been linked to allergies, hyperactivity, schizophrenia, juvenile delinquency, learning disabilities and candida albicans. Read the books recommended in the appendix for additional information.

DO INVEST in the *Low Blood Sugar Cookbook* by Edward and Patricia Krimmel. It can be easily purchased at *www.amazon.com*.

DO START a library of cookbooks. They don't necessarily have to be for hypoglycemics. Many good books with no or low sugar recipes are available.

DO TRY at least one new recipe a week. At the end of the year, you'll have tasted 52 new dishes, thus ensuring that you are not tied to eating the same dull fare. It will help you look forward to mealtime, and you won't feel so limited with your diet.

DO STORE your food properly to avoid contamination and spoilage resulting from bacteria and molds.

DO WASH your fruits and vegetables thoroughly to reduce or remove the amount of pesticide residue.

DO BE aware that chemical sensitivities can aggravate LBS and induce reactions in vulnerable people. Paints, pesticides, solvents, gas stoves, smoke, even perfumes and hairsprays can make some people sick.

DO KNOW the seriousness of smoking cigarettes, especially for the hypoglycemic. According to our past Surgeon General, C. Everett Koop, "It is clear that nicotine in cigarettes and other forms of tobacco makes them addicting in the same sense as heroin and cocaine."

THE DON'Ts OF HYPOGLYCEMIA

DON'T PANIC when you first hear about all the foods that you must eliminate from your diet. Keep repeating all the foods that you CAN eat—there are plenty.

DON'T STAY on a diet that is not supervised by a professional, whether it's a physician, a nutritionist, or a holistic health practitioner. It should be someone with a degree or some training in nutrition.

DON'T FORGET that being PREPARED with meals and snacks is the key to a successful diet and a healthier you.

DON'T BE apprehensive about eating out. Many restaurants now have salad bars, making it much easier for the hypoglycemic (just be sure to use either oil and vinegar or lemon juice for dressing). Lean meat, fish, vegetables and salad can be ordered at almost any restaurant.

DON'T SKIP breakfast. It's the most important meal of the day for a hypoglycemic.

DON'T WORRY unnecessarily about weight gain or loss at the beginning of the diet. As long as it is not severe and you are being supervised by a healthcare professional, it's common to have a weight fluctuation when the body is experiencing dietary changes.

DON'T COMPARE your results or progress with anyone else's. Each body's metabolism is different.

DON'T TAKE over-the-counter drugs or diet pills unless you have discussed this with your physician. They can have an adverse effect on hypoglycemics.

DON'T BE obsessive about your diet. The CONSTANT focus on what you can and cannot eat will only instill more fear, stress and frustration.

GLUCOSE TOLERANCE TEST

So you think you may have hypoglycemia. You have all the symptoms. After discussing it with your physician, he agrees to give you a glucose tolerance test (GTT) to confirm the diagnosis. A test for three or four hours is requested when diabetes is suspected, but a six-hour glucose tolerance test is, by far, the most reliable method to detect low blood sugar. The HSF has always recommended that you settle for nothing less than the six-hour GTT. However, for a different perspective please see the section titled "Ask The Experts" for Dr. Baird's response to the question of whether a patient should take a glucose tolerance test to confirm hypoglycemia.

The night before having the GTT, you will be asked to fast after your evening meal. You are to eat or drink nothing until the time of the test. When you arrive at the doctor's office or laboratory, still fasting, a tube of blood will be drawn and you will be asked to give a urine specimen.

Then you will be given a very sweet beverage called "Glucola" to drink. This drink contains a measured amount of glucose. Your blood will be drawn in 30 minutes and once again in one hour after drinking the glucola. For each hour after that, you will give a blood sample until five or six hours have passed. A urine specimen is given each time your blood is drawn.

Each tube of blood and each urine specimen are tested to determine the amount of glucose it contains. When the report is sent to your doctor, he or she will be looking for glucose levels above or below normal at any time during the test.

During the test, you may start to sweat, get dizzy, weak or confused. If you experience these symptoms to the point of being extremely uncomfortable or you get a headache or your heart starts beating quickly, ask the doctor's staff to draw your blood IMMEDIATELY. Any of those symptoms could be a sign that your blood sugar has dropped to a very low level, and you want your doctor to have the lowest readings possible. If you wait until the next hour, your blood sugar may go back up and your doctor will be deprived of information essential to making an accurate diagnosis.

The interpretation of the GTT is just as critical as its administration. Because individuals have different body chemistries, what is a normal drop or curve for one patient may not be for the next. Do not forget that laboratory tests are only aids to a diagnosis, not the final word.

Remember, too, that the test is not for everyone. Children and the elderly, in particular, frequently require another method. Dr. Carlton Fredericks, author of *Carlton Fredericks' New Low Blood Sugar and You*, frequently used "therapeutic diagnosis." "This means putting the suspected hypoglycemic on the correct diet and watching the response. If, after a month or two, the symptoms are significantly reduced, the diagnosis has been established." This procedure can be a less expensive, more convenient and less stressful method for diagnosing low blood sugar.

In conclusion, if you've read the basic facts about the glucose tolerance test, discussed it thoroughly with your physician and both of you have decided that this test is necessary, read the do's and don'ts first.

THE DO's OF HYPOGLYCEMIA

DO UNDERSTAND the purpose, procedure and instructions BEFORE you have the glucose tolerance test administered.

DO MAKE sure the test is scheduled in the morning (no later than 9:00 a.m.).

DO ASK the doctor or nurse to repeat instructions if you do not fully comprehend what you are or are not supposed to do.

DO TELL your physician, if he/she is not aware, if you are on any kind of medication. Some medications may affect blood sugar levels.

DO USE the "therapeutic diagnosis" for children and the elderly.

DO BRING someone with you, if you are experiencing severe symptoms.

DO BRING a book, newspaper or magazine of your choice to help overcome the boredom. Sitting five or six hours is not something we're used to doing. Consequently, restlessness often sets in.

DO HAVE a pen and paper available to write down all the symptoms you are experiencing and at what time.

DO BRING a sweater with you. Very often, a patient will experience chills during the GTT. It is best to be prepared.

DO ARRANGE beforehand to have someone pick you up if you go alone for the test. Sometimes, afterward, you may be weak and driving could be difficult.

DO BRING a snack to eat immediately after the test, particularly if you must go home alone. Eating some protein (nuts, seeds, meat, cheese, etc.) will bring your blood sugar up, allowing you to feel good enough to get home safely.

DO SET up an appointment before you leave to go over your test results.

THE DON'Ts OF HYPOGLYCEMIA

DON'T DEMAND a glucose tolerance test. It is not always necessary.

DON'T ACCEPT a three- or four-hour glucose tolerance test for diagnosing hypoglycemia.

DON'T DEMAND to have the glucose tolerance test if you have a fever or infection. It could affect the test results.

DON'T BE shortchanged. Go over the results of your GTT with your physician thoroughly.

DON'T BE fooled by the terms "borderline" or "mild" in the case of hypoglycemia. Too often when patients hear these terms, they don't take their diagnosis seriously. This could eventually cause grave consequences.

DON'T DISMISS the fact that you may still be hypoglycemic even if the GTT doesn't confirm the diagnosis. Laboratory tests are not always conclusive. The conditions under which the test is given may alter the results. The best rule to follow is: don't treat the results of the test, treat the symptoms.

EDUCATION: A MUST

Let's pretend it's your husband's birthday and you want to surprise him with his favorite meal, veal cordon bleu. It has been a while since you last made it. You have all the ingredients but just don't remember how to make the stuffing. Now you did have an excellent cookbook—in fact, that's where you got the instructions the first time. You'd better find it.

Your anniversary arrives and you can't believe your eyes. You're overwhelmed by the gift your family bought you—the food processor you always wanted. You just can't wait for a special occasion or holiday so you can show off your culinary skills. However, after you open up the box and see all the pieces, you wonder, "Will I ever learn to use them all? Does this food processor come with a book? It must have directions."

It doesn't matter whether you're whipping up a gourmet meal, fixing a car, planting a vegetable garden or sitting down to learn how to operate a new computer, you need all the information and complete instructions BEFORE you begin.

You need to take the same kind of care with hypoglycemia. Read every book you can get your hands on that discusses the subject. Some will contradict each other; others will be confusing and difficult to understand. No matter, you will learn something from each of them. Remember, too, you don't have to read the thick books all at once. You can read them a chapter, a page or a few paragraphs at a time. Just do it consistently. Learning takes time, energy, patience, and commitment. Don't give up. Just do it gradually and consistently. Don't say you don't have the time or ability—you do.

I wish I could personally introduce you to two HSF members who have taken "don't" out of their vocabulary. First there's Walter. Speak of determination! Here is a man who traveled for more than two and a half hours—EACH WAY—to attend our meetings. Walter was not sure how many miles he traveled because he had to drive very slowly. Otherwise, his 1970 Ford pickup truck might not make it. When I asked him why he made the trip every month, he didn't hesitate to respond, "Because I want to get better. I believe the meetings help me just like Weight Watchers helped my wife. Also, I have a lousy memory, so it's a reminder of what I have to do."

Then there's Hazel. I think she attended almost every meeting the HSF held.

I asked Hazel to share with you why she attended almost every meeting. "I was in terrible condition," she replied, "almost ready to commit suicide. In fact, at one point, I had a knife to my wrist. I threw it down and cried to my husband...he had to get me to a doctor. I was confused, depressed, shaky. I was so angry because I couldn't do what I wanted to.

"I found a doctor in Beverly Hills. He took a glucose tolerance test but stopped it in the fourth hour because I was passing out. He was the first to tell me I was hypoglycemic but that I shouldn't worry. He recommended that I just eat candy, hard sour balls every hour, and go to see a psychiatrist. He also handed me the usual one-page diet. I locked myself in the house for a month. I didn't get off the couch. Then one day I read your article in *The Miami Herald*. Since the diet the doctor gave me wasn't working and I was desperate, I attended the first HSF meeting."

I asked Hazel what the meetings had done for her. "They gave me the courage to stay on the diet," she said. "When I missed a meeting, I found that I would slip off my diet. I also learned something new every time I attended, even if it was only one thing. Sometimes I think I'm well and can do it alone, and then realize that I need support. You not only learn from each other, but you realize you're not alone."

It's not so important what method you use. Books, tapes, lectures—they all give you the opportunity to learn, listen and share. Both Hazel and Walter can attest to this. I hope that one day you will too.

THE DO's OF HYPOGLYCEMIA

DO EDUCATE yourself about hypoglycemia. It is a MUST in order to control your symptoms and make the healing process as painless as possible. I cannot stress enough that **knowledge and understanding of the causes, effects and treatment of this condition are imperative.**

DO START by getting a small library of books—at least three—by leading authorities in the field of hypoglycemia. (See the list of recommended books in the appendix.) Then make it a habit to reread them occasionally. You may find it more enlightening and informative on the second or third reading.

DO BUY yourself a highlighter and, while reading, mark any sentence that you feel applies to you and that you want to remember for future reference. Perhaps there is a sentence or paragraph that upsets or confuses you. Mark it and discuss it with your physician or a healthcare professional working with hypoglycemic patients. Usually, just a simple explanation clears the way to a healthier you.

DO REALIZE that NO book will supply ALL the answers. Some, in fact, will be contradictory. Do take the information you feel you understand and apply it to yourself individually.

DO CONSIDER CD's. For those who abhor the idea of reading or who cannot read, for whatever reason, there are CD's available on hypoglycemia. These, fortunately, can be played anywhere, at any time that's convenient.

DO YOU suspect that your child, husband, wife, coworker or friend is hypoglycemic? Are they reluctant to read any books or listen to CD's? If So get some brief articles on the subject and leave them around the house, office or in their room. The bathroom mirror or the refrigerator door is an excellent place to start.

DO ATTEND meetings, lectures and seminars NOT ONLY on hypoglycemia, but on any health-related subject. Since most illnesses, such as heart disease, cancer, arthritis, diabetes, schizophrenia, are now being linked to improper diet, you are likely to get nutritional advice at any meeting you attend.

DO YOUR homework. Find out about such meetings through your local newspaper, radio stations, TV (some early morning shows will list meetings), cable television, library, physician, health food store, hospital and Chamber of Commerce.

DO CONTACT your hospital, library or school. If no health-related meetings are scheduled, particularly on hypoglycemia, request that they consider the subject. This will alert your area to the needs and wants of the community.

DO WRITE down the date and time of the meeting, put it on your calendar, make arrangements with babysitters, drivers and family members. Explain how important your attendance is at these meetings, and prepare to swap services so that feelings of guilt or imposition do not arise.

DO TAKE your spouse or an immediate family member with you. It will take some of the pressure off the relationship if they understand the causes of your symptoms.

DO USE this time to share. If at first you're uncomfortable, try again at another meeting. Sharing experiences often relieves tension and fear, two emotions that can impede progress.

DO HAVE questions ready. Most meetings are followed by a question-and-answer period. Take advantage of this opportunity to gain invaluable information.

DO CONSIDER attending OA (Overeaters Anonymous) or AA (Alcoholics Anonymous). Even though they may not provide nutritional information per se, they will help you deal with addictive behavior. As hypoglycemics, we are addicted to certain foods—white sugar and white flour are the biggest culprits.

DO FORM your own support group if nothing else is available. Two, three or four people gathered together, sharing and offering hope, can be the best medicine any doctor could prescribe.

THE DON'Ts OF HYPOGLYCEMIA

DON'T PASS up any opportunity to help make the journey back to health through information obtained at meetings, lectures and seminars.

DON'T GIVE repeated excuses such as: I can't drive at night, it's too far, I can't get a babysitter, etc. Perhaps the first time these excuses might be valid, but you should prepare for the next time.

DON'T SURROUND the speaker before or after the program and try to get a diagnosis. Not only is it unfair to the speaker, but it can do you harm. It is impossible to make a diagnosis without a complete medical history and list of symptoms.

ARE VITAMINS NECESSARY?

In 1984, I decided to leave my business partner, Marie, to give more time to the HSF. Our business was at the peak of its success. She and my husband were appalled that I would bow out, but I knew it was something I had to do.

When we were at the lawyer's office to sign the final papers, she seemed unusually upset. Her speech became slurred, she couldn't concentrate and she appeared lethargic. Her problems got worse, and I became more alarmed. Although Marie was only in her mid-30s, she had suffered a stroke two years earlier, and I was worried that it might be happening again.

Questions poured out of me—"Marie, why are you so nervous? Are you angry? Did you take a tranquilizer? Did you have a drink before you came here?" After throwing dozens of questions at her, I discovered the real culprit. Marie suffered from Premenstrual Syndrome (PMS) and was taking vitamin B-6 because she had heard that it could help control her symptoms. She bought a bottle of vitamins and, without knowing the proper dosage, began popping them into her mouth like gumdrops. She was overdosing on her vitamins.

In her effort to relieve pain, Marie, like so many of us, didn't bother to ask questions. She didn't take into consideration the proper dosage, the risk of allergic reactions, and the possible side-effects of combining medications with other vitamins or food. So desperate in her attempt to find a fast-and-easy cure, she did not even consider the potentially harmful consequences. Marie's poor judgment and inadequate information left her with an apprehensive and fearful decision about ever taking vitamins again.

This story is not unique. Situations similar to Marie's occur much too often. They breed controversy. Therefore, for every published article you read recommending the use of vitamins, be assured you will find a contrary view that discards them as nonessential.

The American Medical Association and the American Dietetic Association claim that if one consumes food from the four basic food groups and obtains the Recommended Daily Allowance (RDA), then the use of vitamins is unnecessary. But who always eats a balanced diet?

Both associations feel that most Americans can and should get all the nutrients they need to be healthy from food rather than supplements. I don't think any advocate of supplements would disagree. However, what most Americans CAN and SHOULD do are not necessarily what they ARE doing. In fact, due to certain circumstances, which I'll soon discuss, most Americans are nutritionally STARVED!! How? Read on.

Many of you have asked the question, "Do I need vitamins?" only to be told to just eat balanced meals. According to television commercials, one would tend to believe that a balanced meal consists of a hamburger, French fries and a coke.

Most of us are on a merry-go-round. Not the one for fun, but a merry-go-round of life; one that leaves us too busy and tired to get off and catch our breath. Many of us are faced with job and financial insecurities, family and marital difficulties, sickness, casualties and even death. It's no wonder that little time is spent on learning about the effects of poor dietary habits. Consequently, the diet of the 21st Century often consists of fast foods, heavily fried, sugar-laden, canned, frozen or leftover meals. Here lies just one of the many reasons why most people do not get sufficient amounts of vitamins and minerals in their diets.

Let's take into consideration some of the other vitamin "robbers":

◀ air pollution

◀ alcohol

◀ caffeine (coffee and soft drinks)

◀ food additives, preservatives and food coloring

◀ food processing

◀ medication (diet pills, diuretics, laxatives)

◀ menstruation

◀ soil depletion

◀ stress (mental or physical)

◀ tobacco

Examine the above list and review your dietary habits to see if you are eating a variety of fresh foods. Does your list include fresh vegetables, lean meats, whole grains and fiber?

What cooking methods do you use? Do you broil, steam or bake? How do you store your foods, particularly fruits and vegetables? All of these factors play a role in determining the amount of vitamins and minerals one actually consumes.

So now, where does all this leave the hypoglycemic? Every book I've read on hypoglycemia and every doctor I've worked with over the past 30+ years recommends vitamin and mineral supplementation for hypoglycemics. Vitamin therapy—in conjunction with proper diet, exercise and reduction of stress—has a positive, supportive and therapeutic effect in the treatment of hypoglycemia.

However, before you swallow that capsule, pill or liquid, read the following do's and don'ts.

THE DO's OF HYPOGLYCEMIA

DO BE informed and seek professional advice before starting any long-term, extensive vitamin therapy.

DO CHECK out your local osteopathic physician, chiropractor, nutritionist or dietitian if your present medical physician cannot supply you with this information. The aforementioned professionals are more likely to incorporate vitamin therapy as an adjunct to the healing process. Make sure the person you consult is licensed. Also try to speak to someone who has already used the practitioner's services and thus can give you insight into their ethics, reputation and success.

DO INFORM your physician if you are taking vitamins, especially if you are under that doctor's care for a particular disease or condition and/or are taking medication. Some vitamins and medications don't mix well and destroy or weaken each other's effects.

DO CHECK out the reputation of the vitamin store where you purchase your vitamins, especially if you're purchasing them without professional guidance. Ask questions about the vitamin or vitamins you are considering, such as: What is the vitamin supposed to do? Should you expect side effects? How long should you take the vitamin? Is there any literature available on the product?

DO MAKE absolutely certain that the salesperson's first interest is in your health and safety and not in making a sale. If the salesperson has a forceful approach, leave and look for another store.

DO CHECK the price of vitamins. Once you know what you have to take, shop around for the best price.

DO DOUBLECHECK the dosage you are to take, the time of day it should be taken and any other instructions.

DO CHECK vitamin interaction. Avoid taking vitamins with alcohol or medication.

DO MAKE sure the vitamins you purchase haven't been tampered with. Check that the label hasn't been broken.

DO THROW out any bottle whose label you are unable to read because of fading or damage.

DO MAKE sure the vitamins you purchase are not made with any fillers. There should be NO sugar, corn, wheat or starch.

DO KEEP all vitamins in a cool place, and keep them out of reach of children.

DO TAKE vitamins with meals, unless otherwise directed.

DO REMEMBER to take your vitamins with you on vacation and business trips. This is usually a time of increasing stress, strong activity and change of diet, and therefore not a good time to discontinue any program you are on.

STOP taking vitamins if you suspect them to be a cause of nausea, diarrhea, constipation, etc. You can introduce them at a later date, always one at a time. If there is still a reaction, STOP immediately.

THE DON'Ts OF HYPOGLYCEMIA

DON'T DOUBLE up on or take vitamins indiscriminately! They can be just as harmful as medicine if taken without knowledge and caution.

DON'T FOLLOW anyone else's vitamin program. You should have your own. REMEMBER: everyone is a unique individual with different needs. This individuality includes vitamin therapy of any kind, and therefore should be supervised by a professional.

DON'T RUN out and get the "vitamin of the month." Educate yourself before experimenting.

DON'T STOP any medication abruptly because you start taking vitamins. Seek professional advice about combining the two.

DON'T STOCK up on vitamins. Your needs may change. Buy vitamins as you need them.

HOW IMPORTANT IS EXERCISE?

Have you ever made a list of things you wanted to accomplish? I don't mean just a to-do list for next Monday, but a laundry list of goals that you want to achieve in your lifetime. I've written at least a dozen of these lists. At one point, I was adding one lifetime goal every day. I soon felt overwhelmed and frustrated because I knew I could not complete them all. I had to stop because I felt oppressed just thinking about the three dozen things I HAD to achieve in my lifetime.

No matter how ambitious my lists became, exercise was hardly ever on them, or if it was, it was near the bottom. This is probably because I was never athletic. I was born in Brooklyn, New York, in a six-family tenement house with no lawn or backyard. The nearest park was miles away. Skating was the only sports activity I participated in. There were plenty of schoolyards, sidewalks and empty streets around, but that was the extent of my exercise as a child.

Some of my friends are still shocked when they hear I don't know how to ride a bicycle.

My attitude about exercise changed many years ago when I attended a health seminar at which Covert Bailey, author of *Fit or Fat?*, was one of the program speakers. After hearing him talk on the importance of exercise, I was totally convinced that I had to add exercise to my existing hypoglycemic regimen. I was controlling my hypoglycemia through diet and vitamins, but I knew I could fine-tune my physical condition, improve it, tone and strengthen my body if I incorporated specific daily physical activity into my life.

Now, you mention it and I've tried it—aerobics, yoga, stationary bike, mini-trampoline, jogging, swimming, jumping rope—I've done them all. It was not until May 19, 1986, that I started walking. At first, I walked just a quarter of a mile, then a half mile and then, within a month, I was walking two miles a day, four to six days a week. This was a milestone for me. Walking has since given me more energy and flexibility, relaxes me better than any tranquilizer, suppresses my appetite and rejuvenates me both emotionally and physically.

Hopefully, it won't take you years of procrastination before you incorporate an exercise program into your daily life. Perhaps you can't do it now; you may be experiencing too many hypoglycemic symptoms. However, try making that list of goals as soon as you can. Just don't put exercise at the end.

THE DO's OF HYPOGLYCEMIA

DO GET your physician's approval before starting any exercise program. Most likely you will be given a complete physical, including an EKG and stress test, depending on your age, medical history and present symptoms.

DO SEEK alternative advice from a health and fitness expert if you choose to ignore the above.

DO CHOOSE your exercise carefully. The best exercises for hypoglycemics are walking, swimming, dancing, jumping rope or riding a stationary bike. Walking is the most effective exercise, in addition to being the most compatible with normal daily activities. Depending on the stage of illness you are in, walking is the least stressful exercise for a hypoglycemic. Running, jogging or strenuous aerobics classes should be held off until most of the physical symptoms are controlled.

DO SEEK a non-strenuous aerobics exercise program as an alternative to or in conjunction with walking.

DO MAKE sure the class you choose has an instructor who is qualified through both training and experience.

DO CHECK for information about time and date of classes, particularly free ones that are advertised in newspapers or community news bulletins.

DO FIND a private instructor who will give you personalized lessons if you are afraid to start your exercise program with a group. Use the instructor until you are ready to join a group, which should be in a relatively short period of time. Yes, a personal instructor is expensive, but you will only be using that person for a short time. It is well worth the added expense.

DO STRETCH before doing any exercise.

DO SWITCH exercises occasionally. It avoids overdevelopment of certain muscles.

DO A slower version of an exercise to warm up or cool down.

DO BE properly fitted with the appropriate clothing, depending on the exercise and climate. Avoid anything too heavy and tight in summer and too thin and flimsy in winter.

DO BE properly fitted with shoes.

DO CHECK the floor or exercise area for anything hazardous. For example, if you choose to skip rope, make sure the floor is not slippery or wet.

DO CONSIDER a therapist who does body manipulation or deep muscle massage (osteopath, chiropractor or massage therapist) if sore muscles, malalignment of your body or torn ligaments prevent you from exercising. A massage therapist can produce better results than medication, a frequent foe of hypoglycemia.

DO CONSIDER a "buddy system" if you need support or motivation to start a program. Grab your spouse or a friend, and begin together to reap the benefits of an alternative method to achieve good health and fitness.

DO USE every opportunity to increase your activity. Examples: Park in the far corner of the parking lot (during the day only) when shopping or going to work and walk those extra steps; pass up the elevator and take the stairs; and use a stationary bike while watching television.

THE DON'Ts OF HYPOGLYCEMIA

DON'T SET high expectations. If you are leading a sedentary life, it would be unrealistic to walk one or two miles at first. You have to build up your stamina SLOWLY.

DON'T THINK you can lose weight quickly by pushing yourself to exercise too frequently. You'll only hinder any program you are on.

DON'T PUSH yourself to exercise if you are too fatigued or are experiencing severe symptoms of hypoglycemia.

DON'T EXERCISE on a full stomach or exercise on a completely empty stomach either. Eat an hour before exercising to avoid a blood sugar drop. Remember: don't eat a big meal; you should instead be eating several small meals throughout the day.

DON'T WALK in hot sun, severe cold, or other undesirable conditions, such as rain, snow or strong winds.

DON'T WEAR tight clothes, especially zippers or buttons, if you're in an exercise class where you must lie on your back or stomach.

DON'T BUY inexpensive shoes. In the long run, they'll cost you dearly.

DON'T COMPARE your progress with someone else's. Each body is unique; therefore, length and success of each program is different.

DON'T GIVE up too quickly on any program where you don't see results. Be PATIENT. Some programs don't result in a visible improvement for weeks or months.

THE BENEFITS OF THERAPY

You found a doctor, took the glucose tolerance test and it's confirmed—you have reactive or functional hypoglycemia. You begin to read about your condition, follow a diet, start on a vitamin program and, to your surprise, have enough energy to begin exercising. Even though your pace and timing may be slow at first, it's something you've never done before.

The severity of your symptoms starts to disappear. You're able to function—go to work, attend school and/or handle home situations. You should be thrilled. But you're not. You're full of fear, guilt and anger, and the loneliness is unbearable. You cry frequently. Discussing your feelings with family and friends only makes matters worse. Too often you hear remarks such as, "You should be grateful you only have hypoglycemia. Luckily, it's not cancer or a disease you could die from."

No, hypoglycemia will not kill you but, according to Dr. Harvey Ross, in his book *Hypoglycemia, The Disease Your Doctor Won't Treat*, it's a disease that will make you wish you were dead.

Is there anything you can do? Yes. Maybe it's time to consider psychotherapy.

Although the attitude about seeking therapy is somewhat better, there are still many myths associated with this approach. At one time, it was considered only for people who were totally out of control or for the severely mentally and emotionally ill. Consequently, people were afraid to open up, to share their innermost thoughts and secrets. If they did, perhaps some therapist would label them as "crazy," take control of their lives, put them away or do something else equally as bad.

Some people believe that nobody else ever has these feelings so, therefore, no one else understands what they are going through. They fear exposing themselves and leaving themselves vulnerable.

Fortunately, for many, this thinking has changed. Today, it's not "Are you going for therapy?" but "Who are you going to?" Therapy, and there are many different types to choose from, has reached a level of acceptance. Some are seeking counseling to prevent minor problems from becoming major ones, some are seeking direction as to where they want to go in life, while others are trying to reclaim their lives entirely.

If you feel mentally and emotionally lost, if the physical problems of hypoglycemia are too much to bear, if you're ready to open up and discover the "real" you, and if you're ready to deal with all of those emotional issues in your life that you have put on the back burner, then therapy may be for you. Therapy does for the mind what diet and exercise do for the body. It's an investment that will pay dividends for the rest of your life.

THE DO's OF HYPOGLYCEMIA

DO HAVE a physical evaluation and any necessary tests to rule out a physical disease or condition before beginning extensive therapy.

DO CONSIDER seeking therapy when the feeling of "I can't cope" arises. Waiting until an emergency or crisis occurs may force you into impulsive, shortsighted decisions.

DO LOOK at therapy as a way to explore and discover yourself, especially if you are depressed and despondent.

DO LOOK into the different types of therapy available from psychiatrists, psychotherapists, social workers, hypnotherapists and the clergy. Use the same criteria outlined in "Is There A Doctor Out There" for choosing a physician.

DO BE aware that therapists DO NOT have the answers to your problems. One of the things a therapist can do is to help patients trust in their own thoughts and feelings, explore them and follow through in what they really WANT to do and not what they think they SHOULD do.

DO SEARCH carefully for a competent therapist. Talk to friends. You'll be surprised to find that many are seeking their advice and guidance. Then, without prying into their problems, ask questions: What do they like or dislike about their therapist? Was he or she helpful, and in what way? What beneficial qualities did the therapist possess?

DO EVALUATE the therapist, just as the therapist evaluates you.

DO FIND out:

1   where the therapist was trained,

2   the therapist's attitudes and points of view,

3   how the therapist plans to help you.

DO SEE if you can develop a rapport with the therapist. A trusting relationship between patient and therapist is crucial to the healing process. Ask yourself, "Do I like this person? Am I comfortable? Can I relate freely?"

DO REALIZE that the spouse or significant other of the hypoglycemic is under tremendous stress and often needs therapy themselves. According to Dr. Hewitt Bruce, a psychologist in West Palm Beach, Florida, who I have had the privilege of working with both personally and professionally, "No one understands the stress of the spouse or significant other. I believe that more than the patient, the spouse or significant other needs a lot of emotional support. They're not considered sick. They're not considered ill. They're healthy. They are strong. For the spouse, it's sometimes a job to care for the hypoglycemic, yet there's no pay, no bonuses, no pat on the back and sometimes no appreciation. So many are suffering emotionally themselves, and therapy of any kind could be of great value."

DO CONSIDER group therapy. Many hospitals have programs to help patients deal more effectively with their emotions.

DO REMEMBER that in any kind of group therapy, confidentiality is crucial. It is the only way TRUST can be established, thus ensuring necessary success.

DO CHECK out the new holistic health centers for alternative methods if orthodox treatment fails to help. But be cautious of cultists or quacks.

DO CHECK your local papers for support groups that deal with mental or emotional problems.

DO BE fully aware of all the drastic effects of ECT (Electroconvulsive Shock Therapy), especially memory loss. If you're a computer expert, pharmacist, mathematician, etc., even a slight memory loss can deleteriously affect your life, endangering your livelihood.

DO GET a second opinion if ECT is prescribed or even suggested. Ask about other forms of treatment and give consideration to their use. Remember—educating yourself about any treatment is crucial.

DO REALIZE that the end of therapy is not only as important as but sometimes more important than its beginning.

DO READ *When To Say Goodbye To Your Therapist*, by Catherine Johnson, Ph.D. It will help you determine whether you are treading water in therapy or whether you can strike out on your own.

THE DON'Ts OF HYPOGLYCEMIA

DON'T LOOK upon therapy as a sign of weakness. Remember, it takes more strength and courage to admit that you have problems and need help than to ignore the situation.

DON'T CONTINUE therapy if you feel you're not accomplishing something, even if it's only a small change or a little insight at each session.

DON'T BLAME yourself if:

1   you feel extremely uncomfortable with the therapist,

2   you feel intimidated,

3   the therapist seems judgmental.

DON'T GO back if the above feelings persist. Don't give up; keep on looking.

DON'T STOP therapy too suddenly. Give yourself sufficient time for treatment to become effective and gradually, as you grow more confident, wean yourself slowly from the therapist.

DON'T BECOME so dependent on your therapist that you won't make a move without his/her direction.

DON'T PANIC if your therapist terminates the relationship. Sometimes, because of a sudden transfer, career change or ill health, your therapist must change his/her venue. Your present therapist should, however, assure you that they will put you in touch someone just as professional and caring.

"My doctor told me to just eat the candy bar to raise my blood sugar. I'd rather have gumdrops."

—Suzanne 1998

POSITIVE ATTITUDE:
IT WON'T WORK WITHOUT IT

When I first began dreaming about forming the HSF, I was constantly plagued by my own insecurity. I wasn't a doctor, a nurse, or even a college graduate. What made me presume that I could start an organization to help sick people? I didn't have an answer to that question. Yet, there I was trying to form an advocacy group for a disease whose existence medical doctors didn't recognize, whose name most people couldn't pronounce and even fewer could understand.

What was worse, it wasn't even a disease with a lot of drama. It wasn't associated with children or death, and it wasn't even considered life-threatening. As a result, the media covered it only occasionally. How, I kept asking myself, can I make people realize that low blood sugar is real, that the food/mood connection is real, that people can suffer severe emotional problems because their diet has thrown their body's chemistry out of balance?

I despaired of ever starting an organization which could have the kind of impact that would make people pay attention, especially because I didn't have any fancy titles or letters, such as Ph.D., after my name. Then I started to read and reread. My attitude started to brighten. I found out that many other lay people had contributed to the medical field. People such as Nathan Pritikin, founder of The Pritikin Longevity Center; Jean Nidetch, founder of Weight Watchers; and Barbara Gordon, who wrote *I'm Dancing As Fast As I Can* and told the world about the dangers of Valium in a way no medical textbook ever could.

I knew there was hope. I began to visualize my dreams for the HSF. I wanted support groups in every state, a hypoglycemia hotline, visual aids in schools to warn children about junk foods, and proper testing for people being admitted to state mental hospitals, prisons, juvenile detention centers and jails.

What kept me going then, and still does, is enthusiasm, positive thinking, positive people, faith, trust and a firm belief that this is a job that I have to do. It wasn't simple, not at first and not now. But it is getting easier, and it can get easier for you too. The tools, the people, the places, are all there to help. You just have to be ready to receive them. If you can't cope any longer with the depression, guilt, fear and denial that a hypoglycemic confronts every day, then do something to replace these negative feelings with positive, uplifting ones.

Start by opening your hearts and minds to Dr. Wayne Dyer's books on positive thinking; Dr. Norman Vincent Peale's on enthusiasm; Norman Cousins' on laughter; and Dr. Leo Buscaglia's on love. I also favor more current writers like Marianne Williamson, Neal Donald Walsh and Eckhart Toll. Mix them all together and let them be the cement that holds together all the other necessary building blocks of good mental health.

THE DO's OF HYPOGLYCEMIA

DO HAVE a support group of people who won't step on your dreams, who will encourage you and support you emotionally when you're feeling good AND when you're not.

DO HAVE a good selection of positive reading material or CD's. Replacing bad feelings with positive ones is an arduous task. These tapes and books will help do the job when you need an ego boost and no one is around to give it to you.

DO PUT up positive quotes around your house or office. They will lift your spirits and, as a bonus, they'll help lift the spirits of those around you.

DO USE positive words. Say "I can," "I will," and "I shall." Use only positive phrases, such as "This diet is working. It is the best I've ever had." Repeat these affirmations throughout the day.

DO TAKE 15 to 30 minutes every day for meditation or prayer. It refreshes the spirit.

DO SEE happy, uplifting and funny movies. Laughter is terrific medicine.

DO TRY yoga. It lowers blood pressure and relieves stress.

DO CONSIDER listening to inspirational music, whether it's Bach or the Beatles.

DO OCCASIONALLY treat yourself to something special, whether it is lunch with a friend, a day on the golf course, a manicure, a massage, or a walk in the park.

DO PUT your goals in writing. Read them over each day to instill a sense of purpose and direction. This way, you can check your progress and see that your goals are continuing to be met.

DO STOP procrastinating. If you've put off writing that letter, calling a friend, cleaning out your desk or closet or starting a project, do it NOW.

DO SERIOUSLY consider a job change if you've said more than once—"I hate my job." Look into other fields than the one in which you are presently engaged. Learn what the requirements for employment are and take the necessary steps to get the training that's needed for this transition.

DO SEEK intellectual stimulation. It enhances the body's immune function and helps increase your vitality. Try reading and/or attending workshops and seminars on varied topics—health, beauty, environment, business, etc. Broaden your horizons and increase your mental acuity.

DO TRY to find a teenager, or use your own children, to do extra work around the house or run errands. Remember, you don't have to be Super Mom or Dad! You don't have to do it all—or do it all alone. Share the load of responsibilities. You'll be surprised at how well someone else can do these tasks!

DO VOLUNTEER work. Many times in helping others, we end up helping ourselves.

THE DON'Ts OF HYPOGLYCEMIA

DON'T SURROUND yourself with people who have nothing but negative things to say about the world and what you are trying to achieve. They'll only make reaching your goals more difficult.

DON'T USE the words "can't" and "won't." Negative words produce negative thinking.

DON'T WATCH depressing movies or listen to sad music when you feel depressed. It will only make you feel worse.

DON'T SEE problems as obstacles. See them as a way to learn and grow.

DON'T WORRY so much about the future or dwell so much on the past that you miss out on "living" today.

HEALTH AND BEAUTY:
YOU CAN'T HAVE ONE WITHOUT THE OTHER

I'd like to mention a special someone who, because of her faith and trust in my work and reputation, chose me to assist her for a once-in-lifetime assignment. Carolyn Stein, president of Carolyn Stein & Associates, is a media image consultant. Through her workshops, seminars and keynote speaking engagements, she teaches people how they can create an image of success and develop top communication skills.

Every four years, from 1988 to 2004, Carolyn had been given a very special assignment—media image consultant to the Republican National Convention. For the 1992 to 2000 conventions, I went along as her assistant.

Carolyn and I met through the Florida's Speaker's Association, where she and I were both directors. She soon became aware of my previous work in the beauty industry and that I now devoted most of my time and energy to the HSF. It didn't take much persuasion, though, for Carolyn to convince me to go along as her assistant on what was indeed going to be the ultimate "special assignment."

The Republican Conventions I took part in with Carolyn were held in August 1992, in Houston, Texas; August 1996, in San Diego, California; and August 2000, in Philadelphia, Pennsylvania.

Looking back, it's mind boggling to think that I had the honor and pleasure of meeting four Presidents and First Ladies, including the Vice President, the Presidents' Cabinet members, Senators, and Representatives from all over the country. Added to that list were stars such as Tanya Tucker, Wynonna Judd, Gerald McRaney, the Gatlin Brothers, Roger Staubach, and Lee Greenwood. At the last convention in Philadelphia, the Rock, Bo Derek, and Rick Schroeder headed the star-studded list.

But it wasn't just our country's leaders or the star-studded list of celebrities that I found so intriguing. It was the participation of today's youth, a large number of very young individuals who weren't home "trying to find themselves" or just hanging out with friends. They were here en force, with a statement. They wanted to get involved.

Equally impressive were the senior citizens who turned out. Rather than sitting at home in front of the television, complaining about what is happening in the world, they too joined in and took a stand for what they believed in.

So these two generations, along with everyone else, shed their jeans and overalls for dresses, slacks, shirts, and ties. They put on the outfit to suit the occasion and dove in.

This feeling is beyond politics. It's the very essence of being involved in life and your surroundings. When you commit yourself to life, health and beauty follows. You'll accept nothing less.

I have so many memories and stories of this time. However, one stands out. One evening I was standing in a corridor when I heard a group coming towards me. They were Secret Service Agents, and President Ronald Reagan was with them. Before I knew it, President Reagan was standing in front of me, and I was shaking his hand and talking to him! Don't ask me what I said and what he replied. I was so awe-struck that I don't remember. But I do remember his presence, his stature, and his demeanor—a giant in history.

There I was, Roberta Ruggiero. Whether I was meeting leaders of the world, applying make-up, redoing a hairstyle or straightening out a jacket or tie, I was taking part in American history. It was phenomenal!

However, I kept asking myself, "Why me? Why had I been chosen for this assignment?" Particularly since most of my work is in the health field. Well, ask a question and, if you stop long enough to listen, there's always an answer.

I have repeatedly said health and beauty go hand and hand. You can't have one without the other. So there I was, right smack in the middle of proving my theory correct. Everyone with whom I came in contact had a "glow."

I saw skin, hair and nails—all the picture of health. I felt energy, vitality and excitement emanating from everyone. It was evident that the health, beauty, honor, and pride of each individual present would be a contributing factor to the success of these conventions.

The experiences I had in Houston, San Diego and Philadelphia confirm what I have been saying all along—diet ALONE does not control low blood sugar symptoms. Besides individualizing your diet to meet your particular needs, you must look into a vitamin program, exercise regimen, and stress reduction techniques. You need to maintain a positive attitude, associate with positive people, and look to meditation and prayer for an inner source of peace and fulfillment.

And last, but not at all least, you must look at your physical beauty. It's all there ready to shine. Enhance it a bit with a new hairstyle. Give yourself a facial or a manicure and pedicure. Be daring. Spruce up some old outfits with scarves, pins, fashion earrings or belts. Buy that wild tie you've always wanted or the boots you felt too embarrassed to wear.

Health and beauty walk hand in hand. It's so important to look it, feel it, and be it. Combine the two and you never know where it will take you. It took me to three conventions!

THE DO's OF HYPOGLYCEMIA

DO REMEMBER this section is to spur you on; to start the wheels going and your enthusiasm flowing. It is just a prerequisite for you to look further into whatever area sparks your interest.

DO SET a special "beauty" time aside each week just for you. A time to focus and enjoy the art of taking care of your personal needs. A time to pamper yourself from head to toe. You've been worried about what you put INSIDE your body; it's now time to take care of your outward appearance.

DO BUY some books or magazines on beauty. They will give you more in-depth explanations of the areas I've highlighted in the following do's and don'ts. If money is a problem, spend some time at your local library. They usually have the most up-to-date beauty publications.

DO START your beauty session with a long, relaxing bath. Light some candles, burn some incense and put on some soft music. Let this be some private time just for you.

DO TRY some aromatherapy in the bath. According to aromatherapist Gerri Whidden, "Aromatherapy is the use of natural plant essence to produce health, beauty and wellbeing. A few drops of the essences called Essential Oils can be used for inhalation in a bath or as massage oil to stimulate, sedate or uplift."

DO TRY a loofah scrub brush, and use it after soaking in the bath. Wet the loofah with soap and, using a circular motion, massage your skin. It'll remove dry, dead cells and make your skin feel soft as silk. The loofah scrubs are inexpensive and can be purchased at your local beauty supply or drug store.

DO GIVE yourself a manicure after a bath or shower. Your cuticles will be soft and easier to push back. First, file your nails GENTLY with an emery board. Take your time to acquire the shape you desire. Make sure that you don't file too much into the nail corners. This weakens the nail.

DO PUSH back your cuticles GENTLY and do not use a nail file. Use an orange wood stick. It is even better to cushion the end of the stick with a little cotton. This will allow you to put pressure on the cuticle yet not cause any pain or injury.

DO INVEST in a pumice stone especially designed for the tip of the nail. This will smooth the nail and give you a better looking manicure. Again, this is inexpensive and can be purchased at your local beauty supply store or drug store.

DO TRIM excess cuticles and hangnails CAREFULLY with a cuticle nipper.

DO MASSAGE your hands with cream. Wipe off the cream that is on the nails. This can be done by using a cotton-ended orange wood stick which has been dipped in polish remover. Go over the nail gently, and remove any excess cream or polish.

DO APPLY a base coat. This is absolutely necessary for the nail polish to adhere to the nail. Otherwise, your polish will start to wear off immediately. Then apply two thin coats of your desired color of polish. WAIT as long as you can before applying a top coat. If all these coats of polish are put on without allowing them time to dry between coats, your polish will NEVER fully set.

DO APPLY a soft new shade or try a wild romantic color on your nails, even if you've never done it before. I promise it'll perk you up!

DO GIVE yourself a pedicure using the same steps as above.

DO TREAT yourself to a professional manicure and pedicure. Your birthday or anniversary is the perfect time to indulge yourself.

DO TREAT yourself to a professional facial by a licensed aesthetician at least once or twice a year. In between, a minimum of once a month, give yourself a home facial.

DO START by choosing the best facial products for you. It's very hard to recommend a product but, again, a licensed aesthetician would be able to help you decide what's best for your skin type and tone. If an aesthetician is not available in your area, go to a cosmetic counter at your nearest department store.

DO START with a cleanser that will remove all residue as the first step of your facial.

DO FOLLOW it with a deep pore cleanser. Remember to be very gentle with your skin. Don't pull or push it.

DO USE a gentle mask specially chosen for your skin type. Rinse thoroughly. The rinsing process is extremely important. Gently pat dry and use a protective day or night cream.

DO REMEMBER that consistency is of the utmost importance. Continually starting and stopping any program on health or beauty is most deleterious to your body. It sends mixed signals and can cause undue stress.

DO SERIOUSLY consider a make-up session with a professional cosmetologist. It will enhance your appearance and do wonders for your morale.

DO BE aware that, according to research, cosmetic allergies can also lead to hay fever and asthma. Discuss this with your physician if you feel this may apply to you.

DO CONSIDER a hair removal process, either waxing or electrolysis, if excess facial or bikini hair is a source of discomfort or embarrassment.

DO CONSULT a licensed aesthetician in your area for a professional evaluation.

DO CONSIDER a professional massage. Massage Therapist Judith McBride, R.N., L.M.T., says, "It is my experience that massage therapy is an excellent way to help nurture and heal others. I have found that by restoring balance through the physical being, the mental, emotional and spiritual self are positively influenced. As a Nurse Massage Therapist, I have effectively blended several disciplines to serve as a natural method for wellness by facilitating healthier lifestyle choices and illness/injury prevention."

DO BE aware that the benefits of Massage Therapy include deep relaxation and stress reduction, relief in muscle tension and stiffness, increase in circulation of both blood and lymph fluids and an overall increase in flexibility and coordination.

DO CONSIDER a new hairstyle—sometimes a new look is a great image booster and morale energizer. However, remind your hairstylist that you do want a hairstyle that is simple, uncomplicated and requires light maintenance.

DO TALK to your hairstylist about a permanent. This can add fullness, body and manageability to flyaway, baby-fine or coarse hair.

DO CONSIDER cosmetic dentistry—bonding or veneer covering if the appearance of your teeth is causing you shame and embarrassment—or even if you just want to improve your appearance. Seek out professional advice from your local dentist.

DO BUY a new item for your wardrobe—a shirt, a blouse, a new tie. Be daring—buy and wear what you've always wanted to wear but were too afraid or ashamed to try. Do it—do it now!

DO PUT sleep high on your priority list. It's extremely imperative to get a sufficient amount of sleep. It is during the sleep period that the healing process is accelerated.

DO TRY stress-reduction techniques when falling asleep is difficult—deep breathing, meditation, yoga, stretching, or a hot bath. Put on soft music, read a book—whatever kind relaxes your mind.
consensual.

*I don't want to die.
Can I die from hypoglycemia?"*
—Dave 1996

THE DON'Ts OF HYPOGLYCEMIA

DON'T SIT in the sun and bake because you think a tan will make you look healthy. You'll pay a price—dry, wrinkled skin, plus an increased risk of developing skin cancer.

DON'T PULL, push, poke or squeeze your skin at any time, especially if you have a blemish on your face. You could cause permanent scarring or accelerate the stretching and aging of the outer layer of your skin.

DON'T WEAR tight clothing, especially belts, shoes or pants. Avoid any unnecessary discomfort.

DON'T UNDERDRESS in winter or cold weather or overdress on hot summer days. Again, we want to avoid severe changes in body temperature.

DON'T CONTINUE using any make-up or skin-care product if you experience any allergic reactions. Consult an aesthetician or dermatologist for advice and direction.

DON'T TAKE too hot a bath or soak too long. It could leave you weak. If you're experiencing many hypoglycemia symptoms, it is best not to take a bath unless someone else is at home with you in case an emergency arises.

DON'T USE a sauna, hot tub or jacuzzi unless you use caution. Please follow posted instructions. If you are experiencing a host of symptoms, do NOT use prior to consulting your physician.

DON'T HAVE hair removal done—whether waxing, electrolysis or even tweezing—during your menstrual cycle. The outer layer of the skin is very sensitive during this time and often contributes to more pain and sensitivity than usual. If you must tweeze eyebrows, try applying some baby Oragel first. It'll slightly numb the skin and help to lessen the pain. This is an excellent tip for teenagers having their eyebrows done for the first time.

DON'T ATTEMPT a manicure or pedicure if you have difficult or fungus nails. See a licensed manicurist, pedicurist, or licensed podiatrist.

DON'T THINK for a moment that all of the above do's and don'ts apply only or mostly to women. Today, many men are removing the barrier of "for women only" and enjoying and benefitting from the combination of health and beauty techniques. Be brave, men—give some of this a try!

> " *I just wanted to say thank you. I have spent the past 30 years wandering around in a daze, not being able to achieve much at all. I have become my own doctor in ways and finally come to the conclusion that I have been suffering all these years from hypoglycemia. I have just started to cut out sugar from my diet and with this small move in just a couple of days I have noticed such a big difference. A few years ago I was diagnosed with severe ADHD and so when combined with hypoglycemia I never really had much of a chance of achieving my full potential in life. Maybe now I can achieve something before I die. Thank you for your help.* "

—**Virginia**

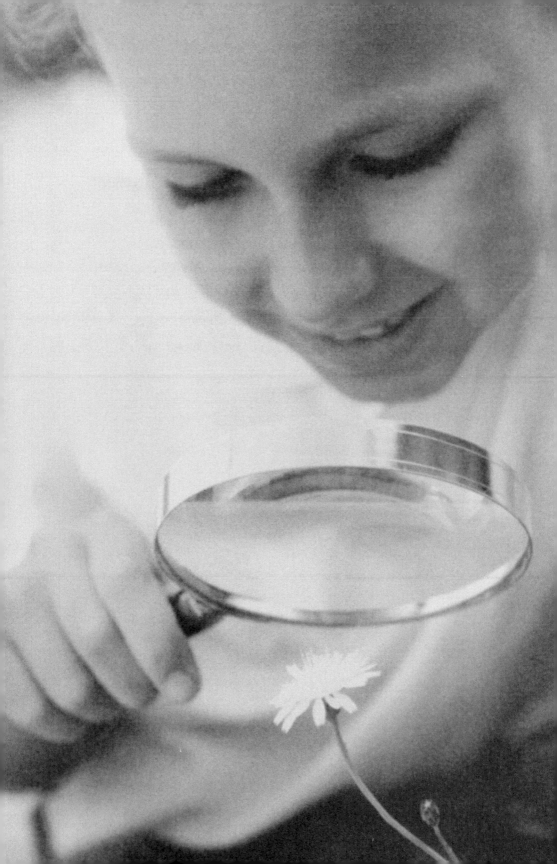

Your inspiration and dedication to helping those with Hypoglycemia has made me feel that there is someone out there that can help. Now my purpose in life is to learn all that I can about Hypoglycemia and get the word out. It has crippled my son's life and almost destroyed our home life. It is that serious.

—**Diane**

ChapterFour
Additional Implications and Recommendations

CHILDREN AND HYPOGLYCEMIA: AREA OF GROWING CONCERN

Since the HSF's website premiered in 1998, I have received an alarming number of e-mails from parents, teenagers and teachers who openly shared their fears, frustrations, and concerns about hypoglycemia. I am including a few of the most notable here so you too can read what these children have been going through. Some of their names have been changed to protect their privacy.

Although their messages are similar, one from Sandra of Cumming, Georgia, stands out. Dated October 25, 2000, it opened with this warm acknowledgement of the support we are providing and a request for more information.

> "Thank you so much for sharing your knowledge and providing a superb web site. There is an area, however, that I found extremely little information and education on and perhaps you can provide enlightenment for those in need. It's in regards to children and hypoglycemia.

My ten-year-old daughter is intelligent, bouncy and happy most of the time. But over a period of several months, she began to experience significant mood swings, excessive grumpiness, lack of concentration, headaches, etc. Her teacher, my adult friends, and my family related her behavior to "a phase," a lack of sleep, or to the onset of puberty. I finally understood she had hypoglycemia while we were on vacation. One episode in particular was a telltale sign. She was having a major emotional breakdown, which was completely out of character and unsolicited, but within ten minutes of BEGINNING to eat, she turned into a person. Suddenly, the light bulb went off in my head! I am so grateful that I did not simply brush off her complaints and symptoms as just life stress or her maturing process."

Sandra had already ordered my book—a good place to start since it is easy to read and understand, even for someone as young as her daughter. I stressed the importance of keeping a diet/symptom diary and working with a healthcare professional knowledgeable in treating hypoglycemia and sympathetic to her daughter's needs. I suggested several other books, particularly, *Feed Your Kids Right* by the late Dr. Lenden Smith and *Is This Your Child? Discovering Unrecognized Allergies in Children and Adults* by Dr. Doris Rapp. Both of these authors, leading pediatricians, talk extensively about children, diet and behavior in these books. I also recommended *Food & Behavior: A Natural Connection* by Dr. Barbara Reed Stitt and *Lick The Sugar Habit* by Dr. Nancy Appleton.

Sandra continued to keep me informed about her daughter's progress over the past year and a half, and she has provided insight into what it's like to be a parent struggling to deal with a child who has hypoglycemia. She sent me the following e-mail on March 17, 2002. No book or author on hypoglycemia could have worded it more poignantly, for this comes from the heart and soul of a mother.

"My daughter is doing very well. We are extremely grateful for discovering the root of her problems. There are children struggling physically, mentally and emotionally, and parents are not aware that their food intake is the cause. I grieve to think of all the children being misdiagnosed or medicated that are truly suffering from a blood sugar disorder. I personally believe that because America is addicted to carbohydrates and refined foods, there exists a huge mass of the population that suffers from intermittent or permanent blood sugar disorders. I encourage parents to modify their child's diet as the first line of action to correcting any physical or behavioral problems they see in their children. It may not be the only answer, but will most certainly have a positive affect."

Looking at this problem from an educator's perspective, Janet of Seattle, Washington, wrote, "I am a high school teacher and have a student diagnosed with hypoglycemia. I have a note from her mother asking that high protein snacks be allowed in the classroom to help treat her condition. However, she eats big bags of chips, drinks soda, and yesterday had a big cinnamon roll from the vending machine. She told me, 'I need it because I don't feel good.' Is this junk food snacking permissible, or is it something I should alert her mother to? She has been absent quite a bit this semester because she has not felt well."

I commended Janet for her concern and for caring enough to seek a solution. And, of course, my response to her question about junk food snacking was—"No, protein snacks do not consist of bags of chips or a big cinnamon roll. This junk food is exactly what got your student in trouble in the first place."

> "Fifteen-year old Randy, from Topeka, Kansas, wrote, "I recently found out that I have hypoglycemia. A few days ago I was at school and I just passed out. I was dazed and after I got up, I couldn't see anything for at least fifteen minutes. Should I have more tests? Should I take vitamins? Please send me additional information. I'm just curious about what can happen."

Randy's curiosity is justified. What if he was just a few years older and driving a car when he passed out? What if he felt lightheaded and dizzy while crossing the street or at the top of a flight of stairs? The possible scenarios are endless and most frightening.

I told Randy that I didn't know why the doctor had not insisted on more testing. This was something he and his parents had to ask the physician personally. However, I did explain that reactive hypoglycemia is a result of improper diet, what you are or are not eating. Stress and lifestyle can also exacerbate it. This is the kind of hypoglycemia that the HSF addresses, and it sounds like this is exactly Randy's problem. I questioned his eating habits. "Do you have a diet high in sugar? Do you skip meals?" I then recommended that he revisit our website and reread "How To Individualize Your Diet." I also gave him a list of suggested reading material and told him he could call me if he needed to talk or wanted further direction.

So where do we go from here? Not every child has hypoglycemia, nor should all children be subjected to a glucose tolerance test. However, one in three children in the United States is overweight. That's 12.7 million American children! Yes, heredity, lack of physical activity, and unhealthy eating habits are all contributing factors. But consider this: Americans consume from 150 to 170 pounds of sugar per person per year! SUGAR and a high sugar diet are the biggest culprits in hypoglycemia. Soda, fruit juices, candy, ice cream and high sugar-coated cereals are the norm for today's children. With preteens and teenagers, parents must also consider alcohol and tobacco experimentation. These two substances, when combined, can be very volatile.

If your child is experiencing any of the symptoms that Sandra's daughter, Janet's student, or Randy described, they too may be suffering from hypoglycemia.

A quick recap...mood swings, severe fatigue, insomnia, sudden outburst of temper, failing grades, sleeping in class, and fainting spells are all possible warning symptoms or signs.

The message is loud and clear. Parents, teachers, and community leaders must all band together to help our children. To understand and learn more about the food/mood connection, start with the following simple do's and don'ts.

THE DO's OF HYPOGLYCEMIA

DO OPEN up lines of communication with your child concerning their food habits and possible associated signs and symptoms. Let them know also that wrong choices, even in diet, may produce negative consequences.

DO EDUCATE yourselves! Parents, it is your responsibility to be educated in this correlation between diet and behavior. What your child eats and doesn't eat directly relates to how he thinks, feels, and acts.

DO SEARCH the Internet, local library, and bookstores, and attend any seminar on this or related subjects. The more you know, the better able you will be to make an informed decision.

DO WORK with a healthcare professional who is knowledgeable about hypoglycemia and sympathetic to your child's needs. Reread the section "How To Find a Physician."

DO WORK with local schools, teachers, counselors and community leaders. Share the information in this section with all of them.

DO CULTIVATE an on-going relationship with your child's teacher concerning diet and behavior. Open, honest communication is crucial.

DO REVIEW your child's dietary habits before administration of any medication, especially Ritalin. Share your findings with his/her physician. Often a change in a high-sugar diet will eliminate the need for such hyperactivity medications or minimize the dosage required. A few weeks or months of trying a diet change first could save years of unnecessary medication.

DO MONITOR the amount of junk food your child is eating. A parent said that his child hid candy wrappers all over the bedroom—under the beds, in his dresser drawers, and pants pockets. This is a sure sign of a junk food/candy addict.

DO EVALUATE your child's eating habits, keep a diet/symptom diary and eliminate the big offenders: sugar, caffeine, tobacco and alcohol. A good place to start is by reading the section "How To Individualize Your Diet."

DO MAKE shopping for food, planning meals, and cooking a family affair.

DO READ labels carefully. Eliminate any foods or drinks with a high sugar and caffeine content.

DO OPT for organically grown and pesticide-free products, especially if your child is known to have food allergies. You can even help children start their own vegetable garden. If you live in a city or an apartment, encourage an herb garden, which is smaller and much easier to keep.

DO ENCOURAGE your child/adolescent or teenager to share any physical symptoms with you. Naturally, if you have a family physician, he/she should also be the first person made aware of severe fatigue, insomnia, panic attacks, fainting spells, etc.

DO REALIZE the importance of carrying a Health Emergency Card with you (or your child) at all times. This is especially crucial if anyone has a history of fainting spells. This card includes the emergency telephone number of parent or close relative/friend and physician. Most importantly, it explains that one is hypoglycemic, so paramedics or other health professionals can quickly administer the appropriate medical treatment.

DO ENCOURAGE your child to share any emotional symptoms with parent, physician, close adult, teacher or school counselor, especially depression and suicidal thoughts. If this is not possible, let him/her know that there are anonymous hotlines available. Check your local Yellow Pages.

DO EAT breakfast. It is the most important meal of the day.

DO BE aware of the harmful dangers in water fasts or diet pills, especially if the latter is taken without a doctor's supervision.

DO EXERCISE. Take advantage of opportunities at work or school to join a sports team, take part in gymnastics. If this is not possible, walk or do yoga to relax, anything that gives you some exercise each day.

DO FORGET the soda; each 12-ounce can has 10 teaspoons full of SUGAR!! Go for the bottled water.

DO CHOOSE broiled or baked chicken and salads if you must opt for fast foods.

DO EXPERIMENT with high protein bars and shakes, especially if you skip meals. Be aware, however, that many bars contain a high amount of sugar. You must read labels.

THE DON'Ts OF HYPOGLYCEMIA

DON'T IGNORE lack of self-control, angry outbursts, hysteria, inability to handle changing or stressful situations. This applies to both adults and children.

DON'T ASSUME that children's junk food habits are something they will outgrow.

DON'T ASSUME that children understand the importance of good dietary habits. They learn from what they see and hear from other family members.

DON'T FORGET to include a daily multi-vitamin/mineral as part of your child's daily regimen.

DON'T PUT your child on any medication for behavior, particularly for Attention Deficit Disorder (ADD) or Attention Deficit Hyperactivity Disorder (ADHD) without talking to a healthcare provider, evaluating their eating habits, checking for food allergies and food sensitivities.

DO NOT STOP ANY MEDICATION WITHOUT THE ADVICE OF YOUR PHYSICIAN.

DON'T TOLERATE any doctor who ignores your concerns or your child's symptoms.

DON'T FORGET to be supportive and HUG your children. Let them know that their problems are important to you and that you will always be there to help.

ESPECIALLY FOR TEACHERS:

DO HAVE information about diet and behavior available for your students and parents, including specific organizations, support groups, and toll-free numbers.

DO PROVIDE in-house educational programs that include students, parents, and teachers.

DO EVALUATE the food, snacks and soda that are available to the children, whether in the school cafeteria or vending machines. Challenge their presence and lobby to have any offending food or drink product changed!! Involve other parents and teachers.

DO BE sympathetic if a child and his/her parent inform you that they have a blood sugar management problem and need to have a snack at certain times of the day. Please don't dismiss this request. A snack can be something as simple as a few almonds or a protein bar. This shouldn't disturb the class or other children. You could even use this as an excuse to explain proper diet and nutrition to children. No one, hypoglycemic or not, needs sugar and refined foods and junk food.

DO GET a written note from a healthcare professional if you suspect a child may be having a sugar management problem. Or request a parent conference and share what you know. They may be at their wits' end, and this information could help them immensely.

Following are three letters I received concerning teenagers with hypoglycemia. Although they are lengthy, I feel that they are too important not to share, especially after this chapter on children and hypoglycemia. One is from a 15-year-old girl who pours her heart out, yet amidst all her struggles, you witness a young woman of incredible strength and fortitude.

The second is written by Matt's Mom, Diane. It brings to light not only what a teenager can go through but how the family is torn apart by fear and frustration. And the third is from across the world and shows that distance doesn't matter. Undiagnosed hypoglycemia still pulls at the heart and soul of an individual dealing with the devastating effects.

I commend these teenagers for sharing their stories. They are stronger than they can ever imagine!

Hi Mrs. Ruggiero,

My name is Lauren and I am 15 years old. I live in Michigan. I was diagnosed with hypoglycemia when I was in the 5th grade.

My parents made the decision to get a divorce that year, and it put me under a lot of stress, especially being the oldest and having to look out for my sister who was in 3rd grade at the time. I started to get headaches everyday. They would last from the moment I woke up in the morning to the second I would fall asleep. I also experienced severe leg cramps that I would wake up crying and screaming from in the middle of the night. All of this made getting through the fifth grade very difficult.

Early into the school year when I started getting these symptoms I stopped doing my school work, and would put my head down on my desk or sit in the sick room in the office for the entire day. My teacher became very worried and tried to make it the best for me by letting me work in the hallway or office when it was quiet, but I still could not concentrate and get any work done. My teacher informed my parents of how my school days were going and instead of taking me to the doctors my mom did not believe me and would only take me to urgent care when I called her from the phone at school and begged her to do something for me.

At urgent care they would only tell me things like "get more rest" or "don't watch TV before bed." At about my 5th trip to urgent care they put me on allergy medicine that I was to take whenever I had a headache. I took this for about 3 months and it had absolutely no effect. It was about my 8th trip to urgent care when the doctor decided that I should get the Glucose Tolerance Test, an X-ray of my head, and an EEG. Both the X-ray and the EEG tests came back showing no abnormalities. When I was taking the Glucose Tolerance Test they had to stop the test four hours into it. They walked me down to the emergency room, where I passed out.

After the test my doctor scheduled an appointment to talk about the test results. They told me that I had Hypoglycemia, that it was low blood sugar, and sent me off with no explanation of why, but with a "meal planning" paper.

I tried doing my best with avoiding sugars and white flour. My parents were of no help and I found what I could on the internet as a 5th grader. I read about what ingredients were sugars and which ingredients were really white or wheat flour, and I was left to decide which foods my parents should or should not buy based on what I found.

I still got headaches on this diet and my grandma suggested the "Eat Right 4 Your Type" diet. This went totally wrong and only made my symptoms worse and made my dad angry with me. I was now in 6th grade at the time. I experienced new symptoms like severe fatigue and dizziness. I would come home from school at 3:30 and go straight to bed and not wake up until morning when it was time to go to school. I became depressed and started to want nothing to do with my family. I became anorexic—I only ate breakfast, and sometimes dinner if my parents forced me to. I was dizzy at school and had a hard time making it through the day after gym class, and spent many class periods crying in the locker room because I was shaking so badly and could not see clearly.

In the summer after 6th grade my dad talked me into going back to the hypoglycemic diet that my doctor had given me one lousy paper on. I researched the diet more and found about the same info as I had before, and was willing to try it again, but I was still severely anorexic at this time. I began to feel better from eating foods that I was supposed to when I did decide to eat, but still got the daily headaches and experienced the dizziness. I started popping 10 to 20 pills when I was feeling depressed. I also had many suicidal thoughts at this point in my life. At this point I did not know what to do and did not know where to go for help. I spent the 8th grade like this too, but made my way past being anorexic on my own and established normal eating habits, and stopped using drugs to give me a numb feeling through all of this.

During 9th grade I still experienced daily headaches, but did not experience as much dizziness as I did before. I had gotten accepted into an advanced math and science center for school, and took Biology and Geometry classes there. I also was in CP English at my home school. I had a difficult time keeping up with the advanced curriculum and extra homework when I had the constant headaches, but getting into a very good college is a very big goal of mine and I tried my best to keep up with how I would reach my goal.

I decided that I was in 9th grade and needed to do some more research on hypoglycemia, now that I was older and could understand more. There was so much more information on the disease now. When I had tried to search the internet in the 5th and 6th grade I had found many sites that said that there is no such thing as hypoglycemia. This is when I stumbled across your book. Many of the sites I had visited recommended it as a great book to start with for people with hypoglycemia. I used my Barnes and Noble gift card and ordered your book online right away.

I could not describe in words how excited I was the day your book arrived in the mail at my house. I could not wait to hear from someone else with my condition that was willing to put their time and effort into something to help people like me who are confused and left wondering after being diagnosed with hypoglycemia. I read half of your book in the first day that I had my hands on it. I immediately changed my eating habits and stayed far away from sugars and white flour and started eating good snacks during school and on the bus from one school to the other. I automatically felt much better and experienced my first day in 5 whole long years that I did not have a headache.

I did not believe that that day would ever come. I am writing you to tell you my story, and thank you so much for putting so much time and effort into helping others and helping people help themselves. I am now able to think clearly through my school work and can be confident that I will be able to succeed in the difficult classes that I want to take. I can now continue my classes at the advanced math and science center and take Advanced Chemistry and Algebra II next year. I also have the confidence in myself to apply to take the Mandarin Chinese class, and I have recently got accepted into it. I also got accepted to take AP Government, which will count for 4 credits in college. I would not have the confidence in myself to do all of this if I did not read your book and learn how to deal with my low blood sugar and get control of my life back.

I do not think I could write in words how much I appreciate everything that you do for people like me. Your book has helped me so much. I wanted you to know that I could not have gotten my confidence back without reading your book. Thank you so much."

— **Lauren**

Dear Roberta:

It was once again so nice to talk to you and share in your wonderful enthusiasm regarding Hypoglycemia. Lauren's letter hit so close to home when I read it. It made me cry again when I think of the struggles my son Matthew has encountered throughout his 23 years and how he still struggles to this day. Hypoglycemia has torn our family apart.

Matt's problems started at a very young age. I hold myself responsible for how a lot of this played out. Our home was always filled with goodies. We were the home where all the kids hung out. Had I been educated in Low Blood Sugar problems, Matt's life and our family life would have been so very different.

When Matt was very young his hands would tremble. I would often wonder if his soup would still be on his spoon by the time it got to his mouth. His pediatrician at the time said it was nothing to be concerned with. I told him we have Diabetes in our family and that was a concern to me. His blood tests showed that everything was normal. How sad I didn't know then. At the age of 9 Matt suffered a seizure. He was taken by ambulance to the hospital and all kinds of tests were done and everything came back OK. We also were sent down to Children's Hospital in Philadelphia to see a Pediatric Neurologist who did an MRI. He told us everything was normal and it would probably never happen again. At the same time we saw a Pediatric Endocrinologist because I insisted that Matt be checked for Diabetes. She didn't seem very concerned and didn't think that was the problem but gave us a blood monitor to check Matt's blood. Matt didn't want any part of it. Looking back we can now see what the true problem was: Hypoglycemia. Unfortunately it happened again. Matt again was taken to the hospital with the same results. Low Blood Sugar was never mentioned as a possibility.

Matt's journey has been nothing short of sad; he barely made it through high school—his concentration was not there. 11th grade was completed with me doing his work. I didn't want him to fail. His senior year was spent mostly lying on our living room floor because he did not have the energy to move. He was told at an early age that he had adrenal fatigue. I just recently found out that the constant fluctuations in blood sugar not only wear out your pancreas and liver but also your adrenals. How sad is that. So not only do you have the debilitating effects of Hypoglycemia you now have to contend with this! In order for Matt to graduate his teachers came to our house everyday to help him thru so he could graduate with all his friends. It was such a hard, sad time. Matt was also an amazing ice hockey goalie with dreams of playing in college. That also came to an end. Many poor decisions were made; Matt took drugs he said because he had given up hope of ever feeling OK. He said it helped calm his anxiety and depression that he felt on a continual basis. His self-esteem was virtually non-existent. Because he didn't do well in school he was made to feel like he would not amount to anything. He always called himself a loser. When you're a youngster and teenager going through Hypoglycemia but it is not diagnosed until later it creates bigger problems and takes a lifetime to regain what is taken away from you. My son who is now 23 still struggles with everything.

Matt had a Glucose Tolerance Test in 2008 and was finally diagnosed with Hypoglycemia. Our doctor at the time told me to write down his reactions during the test to see what happens. There were significant changes during the test. My doctor told us that even though his results could be in range he could still be feeling symptoms of Hypoglycemia. How true!

Matt also worked with a Nutritionist for awhile and was also tested for food intolerances. He had 52 out of 100. The highest that the nutritionist said she had ever seen. Things kept getting worse.

My husband Joe and I spent every other day in school fighting to help Matt. We brought in special snacks so Matt could eat every few hours only to be told that he could come down to the nurse's office to eat. I tried to tell her that a lot of times Hypoglycemics can't remember to eat. They need someone to remind them. It went on deaf ears.

I cannot tell you how many doctors and how much money and how many different diagnoses Matt has gotten along the way. That was part of the problem on our end trying to figure this all out. There were physiologists/psychiatrists/endocrinologists/gastroenterologists all saying it's "all in your head," you have ADD, just get a job and then came the prescriptions to supposedly help all the above. When Matt was on some of the medications, he talked of suicide. It was a scary time for all of us. We spent 3 months at a clinic called the Fatigue and Fibromyalgia Center where Matt received intravenous mixtures of nutritional supplements to help with his fatigue. It did not help and we spent 2 weeks in Texas meeting with a nutritional healer.

Roberta, I spent countless hours searching for answers during all those years until I came across your website. I felt I finally had hope and felt we finally found an answer to this nightmare we were all living, especially Matt.

I think boys have a harder time grasping what is needed to control this demon. Lauren seemed to grasp and understand it at an earlier age.

We have met some amazing people along the way Roberta. You being one of them. Ed Krimmel who you said you met or talked to had tried desperately to help Matt. He knew the life Matt would have if he did not change his eating habits. To this day Matt still struggles with balancing his blood sugar.

I will not stop trying to help him understand the importance of proper nutrition. I think it is so important for all children to learn at a very young age the importance of eating properly. There is only good that can come of it; you would see the bullying stop in school, children would show respect to one another and their teachers and their ability to learn would soar. There is nothing but positive energy that can come from educating our youngsters about the importance of good nutrition.

I love my son with all my heart and will do anything humanly possible to make low blood sugar a thing in his past. Matt's struggles continue to this day. In the past couple years Matt starting his schooling at Trinity School of Natural Health; he became a CNHP at Trinity, Reiki Master, learned Reflexology and Bach. He gained 35 pounds and was like a different person. He was eating properly and his life was looking up. He broke off an unhealthy 2 year relationship and has slowly gone back to his old life style. That is where we are at right now. I am trying desperately to help him again. With the help of his new girlfriend we are hoping to get Matt back to his nutritionist. He has stopped his schooling and the old feelings of desperation are returning to Joe and I. Matt has always helped everyone in his life but somehow does not feel worthy of helping himself. To this day my son still struggles with low self esteem. He has a wonderful support system; a new girlfriend who really cares about him and a mom and dad who will never give up helping him. Matt's Life Purpose is to help others; to let them know there are a lot of other young people out there suffering thru this crazy debilitating disease, to give these kids hope and support that they are going to be OK and they are not weird , different or going crazy.

Roberta, I want to thank you from the bottom of my heart for the unselfish dedication you bring to this cause. You are an ANGEL. God Bless You and the Hypoglycemia Foundation for helping to change so many people's lives.

With great respect,

— **Diane**

Dear Roberta Ruggiero,

I am writing from Italy. I am 19 years old and I have 6 diabetes suffering relatives in my family.

My hypoglycemia is very invalidating to me as I usually can't function well in the morning or afternoon. But feel better in the evening and night (don't know why).

Morning just after waking up is the worst moment of the day.

The worst symptoms I have is lack of memory/concentration, mental confusion, blackouts, cold sweating, heavy legs, fast heartbeat, very cold hands and feet even in the summer, chronic lack of energy, black and white thinking and unjustified pessimism, feeling overwhelmed or suddenly bursting into crying.

My intolerance to sugar is manifested in a peculiar way. Usually after eating something too sweet or just sweet foods for a long time I produce acetone in my mouth and my saliva becomes very acid/fruity. If after that I keep eating sugar I begin to feel dizzy, lightheaded and have trembles. Yes as strange as it may sound I get fainting/lower pressure/lower blood sugar just from eating too much sugary stuff; immediately...not after minutes or hours.

At the same time when I feel lightheaded after a meal and start to feel darker (less light sight) and feel depressed, if I eat something sweet I feel better....as if I was sleep-walking before and sugar had wakened me up.

I also can't stand a just protein and fats diet.

Like a diet of vegetables and fish/meat/eggs...I feel the same symptoms of hypoglycemia when eating like that and I feel the need to add some fruits, legumes, sweet corn, yams...

I really love to know your opinion about my condition. I have been diagnosed with blood works for reduced glucose tolerance but I am not diabetic.

I am going to order your book.

Also I am glad to have found this resource on the internet because here in Italy reactive hypoglycemia is not considered. The mainstream medical consensus is that real hypoglycemia is a condition that only diabetic people suffer from and it's a rare condition, while they refer to the reactive hypoglycemia you discuss in your website as "peculiar of the American literature" and "just a way among lay people and friends to refer to sudden mood change and the lack of energy NOT related to actual low blood sugar levels."

My mother suffers from bad depression. Sometimes she is happy and sees everything through pink-colored glasses and sometimes she is just depressed and sees everything through black-colored glasses and can't see anything good about everything and reason by absolutes.

I can see a correlation between her terrible diet and her change of mood and mindset also because her sister has a severe form of diabetes mellitus.

I would like to help her to understand how her depression may be caused by her diet and blood sugar levels and would like her to read a guide on how to address this problem.

But as I said no doctor or book would refer to hypoglycemia as a common condition many people suffer from but just as a symptom diabetic people may have from time to time. I'd like to translate your book in Italian. I'm young but I'm able to and clearly it's easier for me to translate from English to correct Italian than writing in correct English. I could contact a publisher and make the book available to more people; my mother is not the only Italian person with undiagnosed and ignored hypoglycemia. So many people would benefit from your book.

What do you think of my proposal? Thank you for the time you devoted to me.

Best regards,

— Daniel

"I was diagnosed hypoglycemic about a year ago…I need to get away from the idea that candy and other sugary foods are the answer."
—Stephanie December 2009

HYPOGLYCEMIA AND ALCOHOLISM: IS THERE A CORRELATION?

Alcoholism. No one is immune to it. It doesn't discriminate on the basis of race, religion, gender, or socioeconomic status. Sadly enough, there are also no age barriers. Whether it is used as a chemical, drug or food, 17.6 million Americans are under its influence.

From the womb to the grave, alcohol's effects on the body can be devastating. Its physical and emotional effects can range from upsetting the metabolism and nutritional state of the body to increasing the risk of cancer, liver and heart disease, high blood pressure, and diabetes. It can cripple the emotions with low self-esteem and promote feelings of isolation, rejection, loneliness, hopelessness, and fear.

There is an abundance of literature that indicates that alcohol consumption during pregnancy can put the unborn child at risk for numerous health problems. Even if the child appears unscathed by a pregnancy where alcohol was used, this "healthy" child still has a 30 percent chance of trying alcohol by the time they are nine years old!

Children who make it through high school without experimenting with alcohol, may not resist the temptation through college. And along with the risk of alcoholism, consider these alarming statistics from the National Institute on Alcohol Abuse and Alcoholism, a division of the National Institutes of Health (NIH). "An estimated 1400 college students are killed every year in alcohol-related accidents, drinking by college students contributes to 500,000 injuries, and 70,000 cases of sexual assault or date rape. Also 400,000 students between 18 and 24 years old reported having unprotected sex as a result of drinking."

Information on alcoholism and treatment options is available just about everywhere—in newspapers, magazines, on the internet. The problem is so pervasive and devastating that individuals, communities, and businesses have come together to try to combat and educate people about the disease. Three organizations—Business Against Drunk Drivers (BADD), Mothers Against Drunk Drivers (MADD), and Students Against Drunk Drivers (SADD)—are involved with educating the public about the deadly combination of drinking and driving and advocating for harsher laws for offenders. And of course, the most well-known organization helping people cope with alcoholism is Alcoholics Anonymous, which has been providing education and assistance for years.

It would seem that all the information we want about alcohol use/abuse is right at our fingertips. Unfortunately, most of this information fails to acknowledge the connection between hypoglycemia (low blood sugar) and alcoholism. Fortunately, I have managed to compile a small library of texts establishing a correlation between these conditions.

In *Dr. Atkins' New Diet Revolution*, Dr. Atkins writes, "Experience shows that, when an alcoholic succeeds in getting off alcohol, he usually substitutes sweets. This is because almost all alcoholics are hypoglycemic, and sugar provides the same temporary lift that alcohol once did."

Dr. Harvey M. Ross states, in *Hypoglycemia: The Disease Your Doctor Won't Treat*, "What is most important is the plethora of doctors and counselors who ignore the results of the research that prove that the alcoholic has a blood sugar problem."

According to Dr. David Williams, author of *Hypoglycemia: The Deadly Roller Coaster*, "To combat alcohol and other drug abuse, abstinence, proper diet, nutritional supplementation, and education about abuse and hypoglycemia must be part of the program."

Dr. Joan Mathews Larson, author of *Seven Weeks to Sobriety: The Proven Program to Fight Alcoholism Through Nutrition*, has a phenomenal website, www.healthrecovery.com. Acquainting yourself with this incredible resource is a must! Both in her book and on her website, you will be introduced to Dr. Larson's Health Recovery Center and her in-depth explanation of hypoglycemia and its relationship to alcoholism.

The biggest contributor though to my education on the hypoglycemia-alcoholism connection has been Dr. Douglas M. Baird, Medical Director of the HSF. In our meetings and seminars, Dr. Baird often reiterated, "I have never, ever seen an alcoholic who was not hypoglycemic. It just doesn't occur, it's the same problem."

Dr. Baird's interest in the treatment of alcoholism dates back to the late 1970's, when he became intrigued by the withdrawal symptoms that many times accompany the cessation of drinking—tremors, weakness, sweating, increased reflexes, gastric symptoms and seizures. In extreme cases, people withdrawing from alcohol might even experience visual or auditory hallucinations. These symptoms, he said, often prevented alcoholics from quitting or caused them to replace alcohol with sugar, high carbohydrates, caffeine and/or tobacco (nicotine).

Working on the premise that alcoholism, like hypoglycemia, was related to a faulty metabolism, Dr. Baird set out to design a program to meet the recovering alcoholic's needs. Preliminary physical and dietary evaluations are completed as well as blood and sugar testing. The chemical imbalance created by years of poor dietary habits is then brought back into alignment with implementation of an individualized diet and vitamin therapy. Dr Baird has been using his program for over 20 years and has a 75 percent success rate in helping alcoholics cope with their disease and not fall into hypoglycemia. His program works, he says, because "it stabilizes the alcoholic's blood sugar and thus makes it easier for the alcoholic to maintain abstinence."

The following e-mail was sent to Dr. Baird from a recovering alcoholic.

"I was diagnosed with severe hypoglycemia in the late 1960's. I am afraid to say that I never really took this condition very seriously until now and only followed the recommended diet for about a year. I have to confess that while I was on the high protein/low carbohydrate diet, with the elimination of sugar & caffeine, I never felt better in my entire life. A new relationship and lifestyle change is what triggered my old eating habits.

I happened to notice in your bio that you seem to suspect a direct correlation between alcoholism and hypoglycemia. I also am a recovering alcoholic. While I was in rehab, this was a question that I presented to the doctor attending me. He did not give me any concrete answers.

I suppose the logical portion of my brain would conclude that, of course alcoholism is related to hypoglycemia. How could one drink all that sugar and not have "reactive" hypoglycemia? I do know that while in the grip of a heavy drinking binge, I could almost sense that I'd reach for more alcohol in a desperate effort to stabilize my sugar level and it became a vicious cycle. Try to drink more to keep the sugar level from falling too dangerously low and steady myself from shaking so violently.

I am struggling right now, desperately trying to get myself back on the right path, but seeming to lack the necessary self-discipline. I have even had talks with myself trying to convince myself that this is very, very serious and in order for me to feel better, I have got to muster the determination to give up all the junk that is making me so ill. I have struggled (especially the past three years) with depression/

anxiety/insomnia and I am tired of dragging myself through every day feeling exhausted."

It took great courage to write and share the above experiences. It's clear that in this case, hypoglycemia was not taken seriously. Doctors often don't have the answers to the questions we ask, and many times we have to find the answers within ourselves. Even with self-discipline and determination, this writer struggled every day. I wonder if she/he had the information contained in this section, plus the following do's and don'ts, would the road to recovery have been easier and less painful? I truly believe so.

THE DO's OF HYPOGLYCEMIA

DO EDUCATE yourself thoroughly on the correlation between hypoglycemia and alcoholism by reading *Seven Weeks to Sobriety: The Proven Program to Fight Alcoholism* by Dr. Joan Mathews Larson and *Under The Influence* by Dr. James Mylam.

DO LOOK into the work of Dr. Barbara Reed Stitt, author of *Food and Behavior*. Stitt, a former Chief Probation Officer, writes about her years of research and experience with correcting behavior by modifying diet.

DO SET an example if you are a parent. We cannot tell our children to "just say no to drugs" if we ourselves are not role models.

DO MAKE sure your children are supervised. The greatest risk occurs when children are left alone.

DO GET your child involved with after-school activities.

DO RECOGNIZE the warning signs of alcohol and drug abuse in children: decline in grades and school attendance; discipline problems; changes in attitude, friends, and physical appearance; and most importantly, physical conditions such as loss of appetite, excessive fatigue, and sleeping habits.

DO RECOGNIZE the warning signs of alcohol abuse in adults: personality changes, high absenteeism on the job, low productivity, confrontations at work and home, and increased sleeping habits.

DO RECOGNIZE that most, if not all, alcoholics are hypoglycemic, and unless both issues are addressed, recovery is severely hampered.

DO REALIZE that recovering alcoholics often replace addiction with some form of sugar, caffeine and/or tobacco (nicotine).

DO FIND a physician, mental-health provider, support group (facility if needed), or buddy system that encourages proper nutrition and supplementation with vitamins and minerals.

DO INSIST on appropriate testing (glucose tolerance test, vitamin/mineral analysis, etc.) to determine if you have hypoglycemia.

DO REREAD sections on "How To Individualize Your Diet," keep a diet/symptom diary, evaluate dietary habits, and eliminate offending foods.

DO REACH out and ask for professional help. Medical and psychological assistance may be needed more than tough love.

THE DON'Ts OF HYPOGLYCEMIA

DON'T THINK you can solve your problem ALONE if you are both hypoglycemic and alcoholic. Medical and nutritional therapy and/or guidance are needed.

DON'T BE fooled by the temporary high that alcohol gives you. A drop in blood sugar will soon follow this quick-energy feeling, resulting in the high/low scenario very familiar with hypoglycemia and alcoholism.

DON'T BE ashamed about your addiction. Both hypoglycemia and alcoholism are medical disorders compounded by chemical imbalances and nutritional deficiencies.

HYPOGLYCEMIA: A PRELUDE TO DIABETES

It is rare that I have a conversation about hypoglycemia that the subject of diabetes doesn't come up. The thousands of letters and e-mails I've received over the past thirty-plus years confirm that this is a major concern.

One such e-mail, sent in mid-1998, gives you an indication of what I mean. A full-time college student at Tulane University in New Orleans writes, "I feel like I'm going to die from this thing that grossly interferes with my life...I want to know everything...I don't understand much. Should I just eat everything when I have an attack? Tell me what to eat when I'm freaking...I also want to know how this affects my metabolism? How does it differ from diabetes? Is it the predecessor? What are the long-term effects? Can this kill me? Because sometimes I want to die or just be able to stick an insulin needle in my arm and feel better. Perhaps it is because I am uneducated on the issues, but it seems to me that diabetics have it easier. They can just "get a fix" so to speak. I don't really like needles but I could get used to them if it would make me feel better, feel normal."

On March 16, 1999, the following came from "DM." "I was just diagnosed with hypoglycemia. Can you explain in plain language that I can understand how hypoglycemia is prediabetic? Please tell me this isn't true and if so how could I become diabetic?"

It was difficult to respond to these two e-mails. What do you say to someone who sounds so desperate and helpless? Is information enough? In both these cases however, information is the ONLY answer. When fear and panic set in because of the unknown, every physical symptom becomes magnified. If only they read *Lick The Sugar Habit* by Dr. Nancy Appleton, *Sugar Shock* by Connie Bennett, *Hypoglycemia: The Other Sugar Disease* by Anita Flegg, or *Hypoglycemia for Dummies* by Cheryl Chow and Dr. James Chow. Each of these books would have answered all the above questions! It saddens me that this information isn't readily available through the medical community. Maybe it is because hypoglycemia and diabetes are neatly separated as health conditions—one is accepted while one is virtually ignored. Hypoglycemia is often only spoken of in the context of insulin and blood sugar level management for people with diabetes.

Just scan your local newspaper and magazines. Diabetes (high blood sugar) definitely takes center stage in medical headlines. Right now, type 2 diabetes, like obesity, is at epidemic proportions in the United States and throughout the world. Presently, twenty-nine million Americans have diabetes, with 1.4 million new cases each year. Is it any wonder why this disease is the seventh leading cause of death? Diabetes increases the risk of heart disease, gangrene and limb amputation, kidney failure, and blindness. A leading killer, it also decreases your life expectancy. The saddest part is that 50 percent of those affected may not be aware that they have this deadly disease.

Hypoglycemia (low blood sugar), on the other hand, has taken a back seat. There may be an article here, a book there, but seldom do you see statistics. Too bad, for maybe if we had numbers, more Americans would stand up and take notice of its alarming rise. One book I read estimates that 100 million Americans are hypoglycemic. Unfortunately, there are few formalized studies on hypoglycemia as a stand-alone condition. Therefore, it is very difficult to substantiate these numbers. Often, the only research to be found on hypoglycemia is within the context of other diabetes studies.

Because of this, however, we may never know how many Americans are suffering, needlessly, from hypoglycemia. Do we need numbers to show that there is a connection between low blood sugar (hypoglycemia) and high blood sugar (diabetes)? Or do we just need to read more of the e-mails that the HSF receives?

> "I was diagnosed with borderline hypoglycemia in 1999. My doctor told me not to worry and handed me a single sheet of paper with some diet instructions. Since he didn't seem concerned, I left with the feeling like my condition was 'no big deal.' I kept eating all my chocolate chip cookies and gave in to all my cravings. I am now dealing with the consequences. I feel terrible. My symptoms are worse and I was just diagnosed (2002) with diabetes. Both my mother and grandmother had diabetes. Why didn't I take this more seriously? What can I do now?"

> "I desperately need to find a doctor that knows how to treat my hypoglycemia. My present one told me all I had to do was carry a candy bar with me. My Dad is severely diabetic and I don't want to end up with that disease. I live in the Cincinnati, Ohio area. Please help me."

> "Can uncontrolled hypoglycemia result in diabetes?"

I asked Dr. Lorna Walker, the HSF's nutritionist, to answer the last question. This was her response. "Hypoglycemia is a blood management disorder in which the pancreas reacts to a rapid rise in blood glucose levels by secreting too much insulin while in diabetes, when blood sugar gets abnormally high, the damaged pancreas is unable to bring it down by secreting too little. In some cases, this hyperinsulinism is the precursor to adult onset diabetes (type 2 diabetes). The hypothesis is that the overactive pancreas, when predisposed by genetics, diet, and lifestyle, finally begins to wear down and the end result is diabetes."

No letter, e-mail or explanation can be as profound as the simple black-and-white facts. So in 1998, I added a hypoglycemia/diabetes questionnaire to our website. Due to the increase of questions and concerns about a possible connection between hypoglycemia and diabetes, I wanted to find out if this association could be observed. The goal was to determine whether untreated hypoglycemia is a precursor to diabetes. The survey was also designed to gather information on how and by whom hypoglycemia had been diagnosed and what type of treatments, if any, were found to be beneficial. The HSF received over 5500 responses (3752 confirmed hypoglycemics) from 25 countries!

Below is a brief synopsis of what we discovered. Sixty-four percent of confirmed hypoglycemics (diagnosed by a physician with a glucose tolerance test) indicated that one or more family members had been diagnosed with diabetes!

With this information, we can alert hypoglycemics to the seriousness of this condition, as diabetes will almost certainly be the next stage if left untreated. It is also critical for diabetics to share this information with other family members as a preventative measure.

When we asked those surveyed what kind of symptoms they experienced, the most common were:

Heart Palpitations	80%
Dizziness	79%
Mood Swings	77%
Headaches	74%
Depression	67%
Addiction to Sweets	62%
Extreme Fatigue	52%

When diagnosed with hypoglycemia, only 59% changed their diet. That number is high considering that only 48% of physicians who diagnosed hypoglycemia through a glucose tolerance test recommended treatment. A little more than 50% of the participants incorporated vitamins and exercise, while only 25% changed their mental attitude towards the illness. Unfortunately, 23% considered candy the cure-all for their low blood sugar problems.

Check out our hypoglycemia/diabetes survey on our website, www. hypoglycemia.org. It will give you an idea of what we are looking for and how this information will help future treatment of these conditions. This survey isn't the answer of course, as it cannot take the place of medicine or well-structured clinical trials. However, it is actually giving us the answers we need to encourage more scientific research into this condition that is so often not taken seriously.

Before the future, let's look one more time at the present. Diagnosing and managing hypoglycemia is one of the key determining factors in the subsequent development of adult onset (type 2) diabetes in later life. Diet, lifestyle, age, predisposition, and insulin and tissue resistance are all variables that need to be addressed concerning this issue. To date, there is nothing we are able to do to counteract the effects of either aging or genetic predisposition. The remaining elements, however, can be managed. If one is successful, there is a good chance that Type II diabetes can be prevented or delayed.

Look carefully at the following do's and don'ts. Hopefully, they will encourage you to take action. Making smart dietary choices can make all the difference between staying healthy or becoming chronically ill. In this case, it may prevent hypoglycemia from turning into diabetes. Know that hypoglycemia is real. It is not a "fad disease," as some physicians state it is. It is a blood sugar management disorder and not just a complication of diabetes.

THE DO's OF HYPOGLYCEMIA

DO EVALUATE your dietary habits if you experience any of the following symptoms: severe fatigue, depression, insomnia, heart palpitations, crying spells, craving for sweets, cold hands and feet, etc. See the section titled "Definition of Hypoglycemia" for a complete list of symptoms.

DO ELIMINATE the big offenders: sugar, white flour, alcohol and tobacco. See the section on "How To Individualize Your Diet."

DO FIND a healthcare professional who is knowledgeable about hypoglycemia and sympathetic to your needs.

DO KNOW the definition and warning signs of type 2 diabetes, the kind that we are addressing here in this section. This type of diabetes is usually a result of diet and lifestyle. Common symptoms are unusual thirst, frequent urination, blurred vision and fatigue.

DO LEARN more about diabetes, its causes and effects. Visit the American Diabetes Association's website at www.diabetes.org.

DO FOLLOW the basic diet guidelines for hypoglycemia if you have been diagnosed as diabetic: NO sugar, white flour, alcohol, tobacco or caffeine.

DO WORK with a nutritionist or diabetic counselor. However, be leery if anyone says that sugar and white flour are okay to eat.

DO MONITOR your blood glucose closely. This is absolutely necessary for diabetics. Some hypoglycemics also feel that this is helpful and necessary. The medical community hasn't advocated it for the latter.

DO INCREASE physical activity.

DO CONTROL your weight. This is most important since excess weight makes the body less sensitive to insulin, the hormone needed to control glucose levels in the blood.

DO TAKE diabetic medication if diet, weight control and exercise don't lower your blood sugar levels to normal range. Of course, this is strictly under the care of a physician

DO KEEP blood pressure and cholesterol under control, since people with diabetes are more prone to heart disease and stroke.

THE DON'Ts OF HYPOGLYCEMIA

DON'T MAKE any changes in diet and medication if you are diabetic. Changes must be made under the supervision of your physician.

DON'T DELAY notifying your physician if you feel your diabetic medication has unpleasant side effects.

DON'T STOP any medication without your physician's approval.

"I can't believe my three-year old was just diagnosed as having hypoglycemia. I can't stop blaming myself."
—**Natalie June 1999**

> *Please help! My girlfriend had a hypoglycemia "meltdown" after not eating for many hours. I never believed in hypoglycemia as being a real condition but seeing it firsthand, I'm convinced it is real. How can I help her?*

—**Stuart**

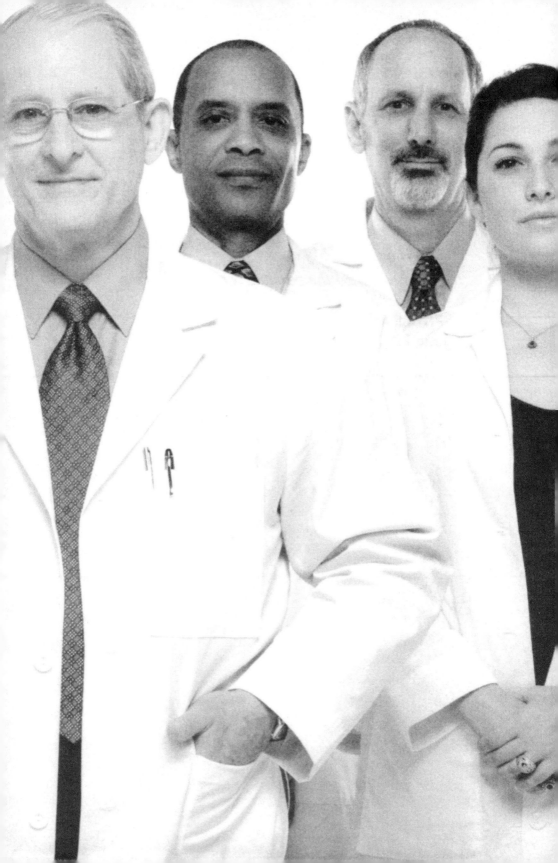

" Thank you about a million times! I literally thought I was dying until my optometrist, of all people, mentioned hypoglycemia —he is one also. My doctor never even mentioned the possibility of this. "

—**Michael**

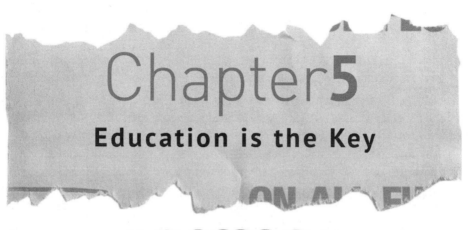

Chapter5

Education is the Key

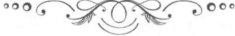

ASK THE EXPERTS

While moving in the summer of 2001, I found myself with 48 boxes labeled "HSF." Since the fall of 1977, I had compiled over 400 files, including hundreds of books and tapes related to hypoglycemia and The Hypoglycemia Support Foundation, Inc. The cry for help was overwhelming. The boxes contained handwritten cards and letters, lengthy e-mails, and notes about desperate telephone calls I had received. Parents, teenagers, boyfriends, wives and husbands all had questions they hoped and prayed the HSF could answer.

And answer we did! Dr. Douglas M. Baird, the HSF's Medical Director, and our Nutritionist, Dr. Lorna Walker, addressed the medical questions. Their dedication was extraordinary. The unselfish donation of their time and expertise went above and beyond anything I expected. I responded also by sharing my own experiences and what I had learned over the past years.

The information contained in these archives is so valuable that I am including it here. I asked other members of our medical board—Dr. Nancy Appleton, Dr. Shirley Lorenzani and Nutritional Biochemist Jay Foster—to share their thoughts on the questions posed to us.

Also contributing are Dr. Stephen J. Schoenthaler, Dr. Nancy Scheinman and Dr. Herbert Pardell. Without their dedication, care and concern, this section would not have been possible. We extend a very special thank you to all of them.

Now here I am again, adding more Q & A's to this 2011 revised edition. Why? Because I feel strongly that this section is the heart and soul of my book. The hundreds of thousands of communications that I have received over the years, mostly via internet now, are a strong indication that the need for information about hypoglycemia is at an all-time high. Although the causes, effects and latest treatments remain basically the same—diet and glucose tolerance testing as the cornerstone of treatment—the stories of the "searching hypoglycemic" have changed. The fear and frustration, depression and desperation, and trials and triumphs are more extreme. Whether one asks a question or shares a story, it pulls at my heartstrings. I know, without a doubt, that each connection I make is not only a moving experience but also a learning experience. This is why I find it so important to share them with you.

So enjoy the added questions and answers. Here's hoping we touched on every aspect of hypoglycemia affecting you and your loved ones.

(*The opinions expressed by the experts should not be construed as a specific diagnosis or treatment recommendations. These answers are offered to provide a framework of information concerning commonly asked questions. Likewise, the HSF does not endorse specific products, tests, or protocols. The HSF encourages each person to take the individual steps necessary to establish the correct diagnosis and treatment regimen.*)

HYPOGLYCEMIA: DEFINITION, SYMPTOMS AND DIAGNOSIS

Q. What is the difference between functional and reactive hypoglycemia?

A. Functional hypoglycemia refers to decreases in blood sugar that cannot be explained by any known pathology or disease. It's a nice way of saying, "Your glucose regulating mechanisms aren't functioning normally, and we don't know why." Reactive hypoglycemia refers to hypoglycemia resulting from the body's abnormal response to rapid rises in blood glucose levels caused by diet or stress. The terms are now frequently interchangeable.
—*Dr. Douglas M. Baird*

Q. What is the most important thing people should do if they think they have hypoglycemia?

A. The main symptoms of hypoglycemia include:

◀ Fatigue and depression so severe you cannot get out of bed.

◀ Dizziness or blacking out suddenly.

◀ Severe headaches where you can't see or hold your head up.

◀ Heart palpitations, sweats and inner trembling.

Since these symptoms can mimic other illnesses, please see your doctor for a thorough examination. Self-diagnosis is dangerous.

If you strongly suspect your symptoms are related to hypoglycemia, start educating yourself about the condition. Read everything you can. Get a few books on the subject, and browse the internet. A good start would be to take the Hypoglycemia Quiz at the end of this book; and then begin keeping a diet/symptom diary. In the first column, list the foods you eat and at what time you consume them. In the second column, list your symptoms and at what time you experience them. Very often you will see a correlation between the two. Take all this information to your doctor and discuss it thoroughly. He or she will use this as a guide and will rule out anything else that could be causing these symptoms.

If all your tests come back negative and your physician is not sympathetic to your needs, please find a healthcare professional who tests, treats and is more knowledgeable about hypoglycemia. Check the back of this book for a directory of foundations/organizations that have referral listings in your area. For more information, please visit our website at www.hypoglycemia.org.
—*Roberta Ruggiero*

Q. I've read so much about the glucose tolerance test (GTT), but I'm more confused than ever. Should I take it to confirm that I have hypoglycemia?

A. Doctors who have significant experience with blood sugar management disorders such as hypoglycemia are able to identify probable candidates for this diagnosis through symptoms, history and examination alone. Subjecting a patient to a glucose tolerance test can be very stressful, and many doctors opt not to do these tests for that reason.

Additionally, the GTT may not provide enough information to establish the diagnosis, which could further confuse and complicate the situation.

A single finger prick seldom tells us enough to be of significant value. It is both the absolute level of blood sugar as well as the change in levels that assist us in making a diagnosis.

Also, the standard glucose tolerance test, due to its lack of flexibility, is prone to error and can easily miss some of the low blood sugar readings and precipitous drops in glucose levels as the patient responds to a heavy glucose load.

If a patient's symptoms warrant it, I use a different protocol for the GTT. This enhanced design remedies the shortcomings of the standard test and has, in practice, identified a higher percentage of patients with blood sugar management disorders. For the purposes of this test, the patient is instructed to eat a diet high in carbohydrates for three days prior to the test. On the day of the test, the patient is to fast from midnight on. Water is permissible.

The first (venous blood, not finger stick) serves as a baseline for both blood glucose and serum C-peptide insulin. Insulin levels are monitored along with blood glucose measurements. The test proceeds according to the standard protocol until the patient begins to become symptomatic. With the onset of symptoms (falling or low blood sugar), blood samples are drawn every fifteen minutes and recorded until stabilizing around baseline level. At this time, the test can be terminated. At this point, the patient should eat something appropriate and should not be released from the examination center until they are perceived to be in control of their faculties. Any examination facility performing this testing should be equipped to manage hypoglycemia convulsions. If the fasting blood sugar level is in excess of 300mg/dl, the test should not be performed.

This test is considered positive for hypoglycemia if the rate of glucose drop is greater than 100 mg/dl/hr or an absolute blood sugar level is less than 60 mg/dl at any time during the test. Whether or not you should have a glucose tolerance test should be determined by you and your physician.
—*Dr. Douglas M. Baird*

Q. Is there a way to do a glucose tolerance test at home?

A. Sorry, there is no way to do a glucose tolerance test at home. Many physicians familiar with this disorder often make the diagnosis by placing their patients on a hypoglycemic diet. If they improve, the diagnosis of hypoglycemia is made. Since the diet for hypoglycemia is a healthy one, I suggest you try eating as recommended and see if you feel better.
—*Dr Lorna Walker*

Q. I get heart palpitations, and extensive testing confirms that nothing is wrong with my heart. My diet is not perfect, but could this be the problem? Could hypoglycemia be the culprit?

A. Heart palpitations can be caused by a number of conditions, and many times, we cannot pinpoint the cause. If primary cardiac conditions have been ruled out (and I assume that the usual suspects—stimulants, allergens, etc., particularly caffeine—have been eliminated) but the symptoms are bothersome enough to warrant additional investigation, hypoglycemic episodes could be triggering palpitations and/or tachycardia (rapid heart rate). Since dietary management is the cornerstone for the management of hypoglycemia, I would suggest that one way for you to determine if there is a connection is to change the way you eat. Remove all refined sugars from your diet, and eat small, frequent meals high in low-fat protein and moderate in complex carbohydrates. Try eating a small protein snack before retiring, but do not overeat. Remember, dietary manipulation, vitamins, minerals and lifestyle changes are almost always part of an overall treatment program necessary to achieve control of any hypoglycemic symptoms, heart palpitations included.
—*Dr. Douglas M. Baird*

Q. I am 29 years old and have just been diagnosed as having hypoglycemia. I have been under a lot of stress and was wondering if this could have triggered the condition?

A. To understand how stress can adversely affect this condition, a little physiology lesson might be in order. You cannot separate the psychological from the physical. When you suffer from stress (real or imagined), your physical body reacts with what is known as the "fight or flight" response. The adrenal glands secrete the catecholamines epinephrine and norepinephrine (adrenaline), which raise the blood glucose levels to prepare the body to fight or flee. Once that occurs, the pancreas begins to over secrete insulin, and the blood glucose yo-yo begins. The drop in blood glucose is real! So you need to be even more diligent with your diet during times of stress. I also believe that once you understand how stress, like poor diet, can set off hypoglycemia, you will understand the need to control both. Also, the more overanxious you become about this condition, the more difficult it will be to get it under control.
—*Dr. Lorna Walker*

Q. I was diagnosed with hypoglycemia several years ago. I am currently suffering from a case of severe hives and am wondering if hypoglycemia has ever been known to cause this?

A. Hives indicate an allergic reaction to something. It is not hypoglycemia, although many hypoglycemics also suffer from allergies.

Although there is no scientific evidence to support it, I sometimes suspect that sub-clinical adrenal insufficiency may play a role in both disorders. The adrenal glands secrete glucocorticoids, which raise the blood glucose in times of stress or increased need. And hypoglycemics respond to rises in blood glucose with hyperinsulinism. Result: low blood glucose. The adrenals (along with the liver and other pancreatic hormones) must then secrete glucocorticoids to raise the blood sugar again.

Some adrenal hormones also serve to suppress the immune system and, in therapeutic doses, are used in the treatment of severe allergies and autoimmune disorders. If there are not enough of these types of hormones, the immune system may overreact to substances normally well tolerated, or "turn" on itself.

You will need to try to discover what your body is reacting to and remove it from your environment.
—*Dr. Lorna Walker*

Q. Sweating along with the faintness when the "plunge" comes seems to be very common with several of us with this disorder, but I don't see it mentioned. Is this common? Thank you. Since reading your book I feel validated for the first time in 30 years.

A. Diaphoresis is the medical term for sweating. People who have shock-like symptoms commonly break out in a cold sweat. This can sometimes happen with a rapid drop in blood sugar, but other conditions can cause it as well, such as a sudden drop in blood pressure or even a heart attack. If you haven't had a check-up in a long time, I suggest one, just to make sure it's your hypoglycemia and nothing else.
—*Dr. Douglas M. Baird*

HYPOGLYCEMIA, DIABETES AND NON-TREATMENT IMPLICATIONS

Q. Is controlling one's blood sugar that serious? I know about diabetes (high blood sugar) but hypoglycemia (low blood sugar), is that a big deal?

A. Low blood sugar can lead to a variety of symptoms, including confusion and fainting. Imagine that happening behind the wheel of a car! Even if your hypoglycemia is not that severe, experience has shown that long-term hypoglycemia can lead to obesity and type 2 diabetes if left untreated. I would consider that a big deal.
—*Dr. Lorna Walker*

Q. Will hypoglycemia go away?

A. Not really. Blood sugar management disorders are hereditary, and as of this writing, we are not advanced enough to change our genetic code. However, hypoglycemia can be managed and controlled. What this means is that with dietary therapy and lifestyle changes, the number and severity of low blood glucose occurrences can be reduced or even eliminated over time. If a hypoglycemic returns to his/her old eating habits and lifestyle, symptoms will quickly return. Also, when we find ourselves in stressful situations, we are more apt to develop symptoms in those areas where we are weakest, with blood sugar abnormalities being no exception.
—*Dr. Douglas M. Baird*

Q. Diabetes runs in my family. Will I have the same sort of problems?

A. Not necessarily. From a genetic standpoint, your predetermined diseases are largely a function of the luck of the draw. The genes you inherit determine your susceptibility to many diseases. It must be remembered that genetic predisposition does not necessarily guarantee that you will develop the disease. Blood sugar management abnormalities, which often manifests themselves initially as hypoglycemia, need not degenerate into full-blown diabetes. These disorders can be managed so that one can minimize the effects of one's genetic inheritance.
—*Dr. Douglas M. Baird*

Q. Is it possible to be diabetic AND hypoglycemic?

A. A diet high in refined carbohydrates can cause the pancreas to overproduce insulin, resulting in hypoglycemia. If this taxing of the pancreas goes on long enough, the pancreas begins to tire and fails to respond with insulin when needed. A temporary high glucose level is produced. When that same tired pancreas finally does respond, it does so with too much insulin, causing hypoglycemia again. This is a hypoglycemic/prediabetic response. If the process continues, the pancreas finally becomes exhausted and full-blown diabetes can be the final outcome. The dietary treatment for both conditions is similar.
—*Dr. Lorna Walker*

Q. Can hypoglycemia affect one's vision, and if so how?

A. Blood sugar abnormalities can affect (and probably do) almost any tissue in one's body. The most dramatic effects are observed with brain function because the brain does not store readily available fuel. Other tissue areas are affected to a greater or lesser extent based on the tissue's susceptibility to blood sugar fluctuations as well as fuel storage capabilities. The eye is an extension of the brain. It is a neutral tissue, does not store fuel and is susceptible to damage caused by reduced availability of fuel and/or oxygen.
—*Dr. Douglas M. Baird*

HYPOGLYCEMIA AND DEPRESSION

Q. I have most of the symptoms of hypoglycemia, especially depression and mood swings. My doctor wants to put me on antidepressants. How can I convince him to take a glucose tolerance test first?

A. Depression and mood swings can certainly be a part of the symptom complex associated with hypoglycemia. They can also be symptoms of other disorders. The common work-up to begin to identify some of the underlying causes of these symptoms includes general chemistries, blood count, thyroid function testing and, if the symptoms warrant, glucose tolerance testing. If your doctor is unwilling to make the effort to eliminate the causes of your symptoms (for whatever reason), it may be time to consider seeking a second opinion.
—*Dr. Douglas M. Baird*

Q. I have a friend who was diagnosed as having hypoglycemia. She feels really bad, her doctor doesn't help and I don't know what to do. She is talking about suicide! Please help me help her.

A. First and foremost, call your local suicide prevention hotline. Every county has one and the number is usually on the front page of the local phone directory. You can also call the National Suicide Prevention Lifeline at 1-800-273-TALK.

Have you talked with your friend's family about her situation? Her family, as well as her priest, rabbi, or spiritual advisor, could be important allies in her recovery to health. You and they should also work to help her find a health professional who takes her situation seriously.

In the meantime, check out Dr. Joan Larson's website at www. healthrecovery.com. Dr. Larson writes extensively on hypoglycemia/ depression and suicide—a must read for you, your friend and her family.

Remember, your friend must be willing to do the work to rebuild her health. All your good intentions will go nowhere without her commitment and willingness to make life changes.
—*Roberta Ruggiero*

Q. I have been diagnosed as having hypoglycemia. However, I am also very depressed. Is this a symptom of this condition? Are they related or am I going crazy?

A. Clinical depression is becoming a more commonly diagnosed disorder as more information becomes available and as the medical profession becomes better educated regarding diagnosis and treatment of this truly devastating disorder. Most of us have been taught that depression is an emotional illness that is best treated by simply getting over it.

Through research, however, a different picture is beginning to emerge. It now appears that clinical depression, that is depression without any obvious environmental cause, is not an imaginary or mental disorder at all. There is scientific evidence that these forms of depression are often caused by a chemical malfunction in the brain itself. Depression is no more imaginary than heart disease or cancer.

Although there are many causes for this observable chemical aberration and because the subject of this book is hypoglycemia, we will expand on the role of blood sugar as one of the factors in the development of this disorder.

The brain is absolutely dependent on a constant, uninterrupted source of fuel for proper function. Sugar (or glucose) is the primary fuel that supplies the brain with the energy that it needs to function properly. The brain cannot store fuel, so the sugar levels in the blood that supplies the brain must stay constantly high enough to supply its needs.

In hypoglycemics, the principal problem is maintaining a reasonably constant and high enough blood sugar level to insure proper function of all organ systems, the brain being the most important. When the fuel supply of the brain drops below a certain critical level, the brain begins to malfunction. The same thing happens to your home computer when the power supply is interrupted or altered. Anything that can possibly go wrong—will.

Any brain dysfunction can and will occur under these circumstances, including (but not limited to) anxiety, depression, memory loss, confusion, mood swings and, in its worst form, diagnosable mental illness.

The importance of correcting or at least managing this critical element for brain function cannot be overemphasized. Depression can be a direct result of blood sugar mismanagement. Both disorders seem to be affecting a significant percentage of our population. Drug therapy, while very important, is only a partial fix. Stabilizing blood sugar levels is an important element in the long-term management of depression.
—*Dr. Douglas M. Baird*

Q. I have been diagnosed with hypoglycemia and am grateful I already see a big difference in my health and attitude since going on a hypoglycemia diet. However, I would like to stop my medication. I take antidepressants and tranquilizers. I don't think I need them anymore. Any suggestions?

A. I am happy that just changing your eating habits has made such a significant change in your life. Most likely you've omitted one or some of the big offenders—sugar, white flour, alcohol, caffeine and tobacco. Whatever your approach, it is working.

As far as decreasing your medications and eventually getting off of them, it is imperative that you work with a healthcare professional who not only tests and treats hypoglycemia but also knows your medical history, the type of medications you are on and the dosage.

I can only share with you what helped me. After my official diagnosis of hypoglycemia, a physician who combined holistic healthcare with orthodox medicine was a huge help to me. In time, vitamins, exercise and stress-reduction techniques aided in my healing process. Although my doctor slowly started reducing the dosages of my medication, it wasn't until I was introduced to hypnosis that was I able to get off them completely. Through deep relaxation, guided imagination and suggestions, and the help of a highly professional hypnotherapist, my goals were reached.

If you ever think of using hypnosis or any other type of alternative therapy, I urge you to learn everything you can about the treatment. Then take this information to your physician and decide together if this may be something you should consider.

Since depression can be caused by a chemical imbalance, hypnosis alone may not work for you. DO NOT stop your medication on your own, and if you are advised that you can stop it, make sure you are under medical supervision while doing so and report any symptoms such as worsening depression, suicidal thoughts or other side effects immediately.
—*Roberta Ruggiero*

Q. I've just been diagnosed as having hypoglycemia after years of being told that my symptoms "were all in my head." I'm not only having a hard time with my diet but with my emotions. I am so angry at all the doctors, my family included, who never really believed that this is a tried and true condition. I'm working on my diet, but how can I get past my anger?

A. The only reason why the people in your past labeled your hypoglycemia as "all in your head" was because they had no understanding of what was actually taking place. Can you really be angry at someone because they have never been exposed to something or because, generally, our knowledge of the disease is in a developmental state?

They weren't making a value judgment about you; they were merely reaching for the only reason they could find. I notice that the solution to a problem does not appear until a person is truly ready to see it and confront it. That is, ask yourself these questions: "Was I really ready to deal with this back then? How have I grown from the difficulty of living with this? Who am I as a result of this?"

Anger is a complex emotion. While it may be destructive, it may also be motivating and empowering. The key is to change the energy of the anger into a positive force. Interestingly, if you do not, and you remain stuck in the anger, it may actually interfere with your sugar. By remaining angry, you may create blood sugar instability. Therefore, via another route, you will allow these individuals to continue to block your healing.

—*Dr. Nancy Scheinman*

HYPOGLYCEMIA AND ALCOHOL

Q. My husband quit drinking and now craves chocolate.

A. This is not an uncommon response. Alcohol is simply a very refined sugar. When people quit one form of sugar, they many times substitute another. I have never seen an alcoholic that was not hypoglycemic. Alcohol and sugar are different forms of the same fuel. The inability to properly manage blood sugar levels in the bloodstream may cause a variety of problems, especially with brain function. This can be quite serious. The problem of proper and adequate fueling of the brain must be managed on an ongoing basis if an individual is to function optimally.

—*Dr. Douglas M. Baird*

Q. My husband has been drinking extensively, and it's affecting every aspect of our lives. He's almost at the point of losing his job, and if this keeps up, he'll lose everything—including me. A friend recommended Dr. Joan Larson's *Seven Weeks to Sobriety.* **I glanced at it and saw that hypoglycemia and alcoholism are related. If this is true, how can I help him and where do I start?**

A. Please read Dr. Joan Larson's book, and then read the section in this book on "Hypoglycemia & Alcoholism: Is There A Correlation?" That's a good place to start. Not only will you begin to understand how these two conditions are related, but I list more than a dozen simple do's and don'ts to help cope with this addiction.

Take this information and a diet/symptom diary to your husband's doctor. Discuss in detail what you have learned from reading about alcoholism and the importance of addressing his blood sugar control. Your husband may be fooled by the temporary high that alcohol is giving him. However, a drop in blood sugar will soon follow this quick-energy feeling, resulting in the high/low scenario very familiar with hypoglycemia and alcoholism.

Also discuss with your physician the benefits of having your husband work with a mental health counselor and attend support groups such as AA (Alcoholics Anonymous for your husband and Al-Anon for you), and address the importance of proper diet and nutritional supplements. This

may seem like a tall order to discuss with one doctor. It just shows that choosing a primary care physician is one of the most important decisions a person can make. Then when an emergency arises (especially since it affects the whole family), it is much easier for a doctor and patient to make life-altering decisions together.
—*Roberta Ruggiero*

Q. Can having severe hypoglycemia give a false (high) blood alcohol level with a Breathalyzer?

A. When one's blood sugar gets too low, the human body has a number of compensatory mechanisms that will try to correct this condition. One of those processes is called gluconeogenesis, literally "making new sugar." One of the byproducts of that process is acetone. This is the reason why people with blood sugar problems and those on caloric restrictive diets have what the medical profession calls "acetone breath." Law enforcement personnel often confuse this smell with alcohol. Now, whether the Breathalyzer can discriminate between acetone, other ketones, and alcohol is the critical question. Your attorney will have to contact the manufacturers of that technology to see whether that discrimination can be made by the available technology. I do not have a definitive answer to that question.
—*Dr. Douglas M. Baird*

Q. This is not so much a question as a statement. I struggled with alcoholism for almost one third of my life, trying everything from Alcoholics Anonymous to hypnotherapy. Nothing worked and I was anxious, depressed; my drinking was out of control. I had two DUI's and was working on a third, which would result in a year in prison if I could not find a way to stop drinking. My parents had given me a book, *Seven Weeks to Sobriety*, by Joan Matthews Larson, Ph.D., and despite my qualms about it, I decided to read it. This book changed my life. The book notes that almost all alcoholics have hypoglycemia and very low levels of amino acids, vitamins and minerals, resulting in strong unmanageable cravings for alcohol (sugar), and due to the lack of vital amino acids, vitamins and minerals, the brain cannot maintain the proper brain chemistry for well being. Glutamine has been an absolute wonder in helping with cravings for alcohol. I am now free of this hell that I thought was caused by just being weak.

Please pass on this information. It is vital in treating this disease. Talk therapy cannot stabilize blood sugar and rebalance brain chemistry. Dr. Larson is the founder of the Health Recovery Center in Minneapolis, Minnesota.

A. Thank you so much for sharing your story. The HSF is very lucky to have Dr. Douglas M. Baird as our Medical Director. It was Dr. Baird who first told us about the correlation between hypoglycemia and alcoholism some 29 years ago. His information was so important and impressive that I devoted a whole section to this subject when I updated my book in 1993. I also mention the work of Dr. Joan Larson and recommend her book and website, www.sevenweekstosobriety.com, whenever I can. It is the dedication and devotion of doctors like Dr. Baird and Dr. Larson that can save the lives of many hypoglycemics who also suffer from alcoholism. We are lucky to have them.
—*Roberta Ruggiero*

Q. I have hypoglycemia but I am also struggling with alcoholism. Even though I brought this up with my physician, his main concern is my liver enzymes. What does he mean?

A. Hypoglycemia often accompanies alcoholism. Your liver plays an important role in regulating blood sugar. It stores excess glucose in the form of glycogen (starch) and releases it back into the bloodstream as glucose between meals when your body needs it. The liver can also turn protein into glucose for energy as well (called gluconeogenesis) when glycogen stores are depleted. Alcohol is toxic to the liver and can impair the liver's ability to perform its tasks. When the liver is injured, enzymes within the liver leak into the bloodstream and are therefore elevated. Elevated liver enzymes are an indication of liver damage. Abstinence and avoiding sugar and refined carbohydrates prevent further damage to the liver and improve hypoglycemia.
—*Dr. Lorna Walker*

Hypoglycemia & Surgery/Medical Procedures

Q. I must have surgery and I'm hypoglycemic. I'm not concerned about the procedure, but I am worried about the intravenous glucose. Is there anything else the doctors can give me instead?

A. Yes, there are other IV fluids that can be utilized in a hospital setting that will not affect your blood sugar. Ask your doctor. The stress of the surgery itself, however, may adversely affect your ability to manage your blood sugar. While this is a nuisance, it can be brought under control once you are back home.
—*Dr. Douglas M. Baird*

Q. I am a post gastric bypass patient. I take Precose (acarbose) before meals, but I am still am having blood glucose lows with a diet consisting of 35-40 grams of carbohydrates at lunch and supper. I am eating only protein at breakfast. Any suggestions are appreciated.

A. Unfortunately, hypoglycemia is a common side effect of gastric bypass (bariatric) surgery, and you'll have to struggle with it until your insulin levels start to decrease as you lose more weight. You may have to decrease your carbohydrate intake and increase proteins during this transition period and eat more frequently. As you continue to lose weight, your high insulin levels should decrease, and you should be able to tolerate more carbohydrates.

It is important to remember, however, that you will have to eat less carbohydrates and more protein than you did before the surgery and in smaller, more frequent meals, for the rest of your life.
—*Dr. Lorna Walker*

Q. Help! I have to have a colonoscopy. However, I have hypoglycemia and need suggestions fast.

A. The following procedure has helped me and others I have shared it with. Make a pot of homemade chicken soup (or beef) the day before you have to fast. If you can't, try to buy it fresh from a local deli or restaurant. As a last resort, buy chicken broth from your local supermarket—preferably in a box and not a can. On the day of the fast, sip just the broth throughout the day. Avoid fruit juices or any other sugar-laden drinks, just drink plenty of water. Rest as much as possible, sleep if you can and stay calm and positive by doing what works for you—read a book, watch TV or meditate—anything that doesn't add stress.

On the day of the test, bring a snack with you that you can eat immediately after the procedure. —*Roberta Ruggiero*

Q. I was just diagnosed with hypoglycemia and found out what I can't eat. Sounds like everything I love. I feel so deprived. Will I ever eat normal again?

A. We often have an emotional relationship with food, turning to it for comfort more than for its nutritional value. I believe we have to think differently about food and its role in our lives.

For those of us with hypoglycemia, looking at it from this perspective may help—there's no medication, surgery, chemotherapy or transplant that can help us. Proper diet is the key to controlling symptoms.

And there is so much to eat. Check out the list of allowable foods and suggested recipes in this book. You mainly have to avoid sugar (especially sugary desserts), white flour, dried fruits, processed meats, alcohol and caffeine. Not a bad suggestion for anyone who wants to eat healthily. And for those of us with hypoglycemia, it helps keep us symptom free!

Education and preparation are key factors. Read everything you can on this subject, and research hypoglycemia/low sugar/low refined food diet menus in the library or on the internet. Ask your family and friends for their recipes, and adjust to your individual needs. Have food available at all times, but make it simple and easy. That's the key to avoiding that deprived feeling. After introducing fresh, wholesome foods into your diet, you'll be surprised at how much more you enjoy them.

Obviously, if these suggestions don't help and you still feel depressed and deprived, seek professional guidance.
—*Roberta Ruggiero*

Q. I am so confused. One book says I can eat whole wheat, and another book says I should avoid it. As a hypoglycemic trying to figure out what to eat, this is so confusing. What's correct?

A. Many people have made themselves allergic to wheat and dairy due to eating sugar with these products (cakes, cookies, pies, pastries, ice cream, cheesecake, yogurt, etc.). I personally do not think a hypoglycemic should eat any sugar, wheat or dairy. The best foods to eat are whole foods, not processed foods like bread, boxed cereals, pasta, pizza, etc. That said, many other experts believe that natural whole grains coupled with protein have a place in the diet for hypoglycemia. The choice is yours.
—*Dr. Nancy Appleton*

Q. I have hypoglycemia and read about the importance of the glycemic index. What is it and how can it help me?

A. The glycemic index, sometimes called GI, is a rating scale for carbohydrate foods and uses a number to show how each food affects blood sugar. Foods are rated on a scale of 1-100. The shakers and movers, those carbohydrates that are broken down and converted rapidly into blood sugar, are given a high number on the scale, usually above 55. Carbs with more gentle blood sugar effects are given a number lower than 55. The index will help you choose those foods and alert you to foods that could shake the foundations of your stability. All wheat, even whole wheat, is relatively high, usually in the 70s. That doesn't mean you should never eat bread. What it might mean is that "woman should not live by bread alone." Don't think that a piece of whole wheat bread by itself is a good snack for the peace and tranquility of your blood. To make that organic whole grain bread work for you, you must add a low index food like peanut or almond butter. Adding a protein will also dull the blood sugar racing effects. Poultry, meat, or fish as an open-faced sandwich might be a good main course to keep your weight and mood in good shape. Use your computer and Amazon to research books on this topic. Your local library or bookstore is likely to have a book or two focused on the GI. There are pocketbook rating guides of up to 1,000 foods and cookbooks that can assist you in putting together meals and snacks. Combining high number foods with lower ones can give variety to your diet and prevent your surrendering some of your favorite items. The website of Al Sears, M.D., www.alsearsmd.com, allows you to download a glycemic index for easy reference. Like other glycemic index sites, Dr. Sears offers a free newsletter to keep you updated and inspired.
—*Dr. Shirley Lorenzani*

Q. What is your opinion about eating protein to manage low blood sugar?

A. Protein is not a "solution" to hypoglycemia. Protein can be used as a body fuel and is digested more slowly than carbohydrates and sugars. It is broken down into amino acids that can be turned into "fuel" later by the body if needed. Too much protein in the diet can lead to ketosis; too little can lead to protein starvation. The idea is to maintain a diet moderate in low-fat protein, low in carbohydrates (but not too low) and devoid of simple sugars. This will help rest an overactive pancreas and help maintain steady blood glucose levels.
—*Dr. Lorna Walker*

Q. What should I eat when my low blood sugar hits? Orange juice? A candy bar?

A. As previously stated, the worst thing you can eat when your hypoglycemia "hits" is sugar in any form! It may make you feel better temporarily, but soon afterwards your pancreas will over secrete insulin, which caused your blood sugar to drop in the first place. Eating small, frequent meals that are low in fat and carbohydrates and contain moderate amounts of protein is the best way to control your blood sugar. Over time, you will learn what works best for you to keep your sugar within a reasonable range.
—*Dr. Douglas M. Baird*

Q. If foods like sugar and bread raise blood glucose, why can't hypoglycemics have these foods?

A. Yes, these foods raise the blood glucose. However, in reactive hypoglycemia it is the pancreas that is the problem. Each time the blood sugar is raised with these foods, the pancreas of a hypoglycemic secretes too much insulin in response and sends the blood glucose spiraling down. Thus it is the pancreas's response to eating these foods that causes the hypoglycemia. If not addressed by diet, hypoglycemia can often lead to adult-onset diabetes. The overworked pancreas tires out and fails to produce enough insulin. The diet for hypoglycemia stabilizes blood glucose levels and rests the pancreas.
—*Dr. Lorna Walker*

Q. I am 18 years old and have hypoglycemia. I've been able to control my symptoms but with my Mom's help. She makes it easy because she cooks everything I'm supposed to eat. I'm off to college in a few weeks and worried about how and if I can stick to a hypoglycemia diet.

A. As you look around at your classmates, you probably see them eating and drinking foods that contain high amounts of high-fructose corn syrup, one of the worst ingredients for maintaining steady blood sugar. Donuts, candy bars, sodas, energy drinks, and flavored water are among the culprits. Don't think those students are getting away with their diet. You reap what you swallow! In that perspective, all of the students are hypoglycemic. Their food choices determine whether or not they are feeling the symptoms.

UC Berkeley sent a copy of *The Omnivore's Dilemma* by Michael Pollan to incoming students in the College of Letters and Science this year (2009).

Students were asked to read the book over the summer and sign up for food-focused discussion groups and classes in the fall semester. One of Pollan's main points is that our Homo sapiens brain evolved to a large size because we require a lot of brainpower to make wise food choices. Just because a food is sold in the grocery store or college cafeteria doesn't mean it can sustain your health. He asserts that health can be built and nurtured by being informed about foods and what they do to your body. Simple, whole foods are usually the best choice. That usually works for hypoglycemia as well as other health challenges.

After you make your move to college, explore nearby grocery stores, farmers' markets, and restaurants to find foods similar to what your mom has been cooking for you at home. Maybe you can improve on what your mom has done! You are considered an adult by the military, voting registrar, the bars in many states, and law enforcement. It's time to assert the responsibility for your blood sugar levels.

If you don't have a kitchen available, and it's permitted in your living situation, invest in a hot plate, crock pot, and mini-fridge. This way you can easily cook healthy basics like beans, quinoa, fresh vegetables, meat, poultry, eggs, and fish. If you have to rely on your school's cafeteria food, be assertive in making suggestions to the manager. Chances are other students feel the same way you do, and your activism will be appreciated.
—*Dr. Shirley Lorenzani*

Q. I've been having more trouble with my low blood sugar lately. I was wondering if there was a dietary way to get back to normal after a bout of very low blood sugar (near passing out). I know I need some juice at first, but what is the next best thing I should be eating after that and for the rest of the day?

A. Try not to respond to drops in blood sugar with sugar such as that found in juice. It only continues the cycle of highs and lows. If you must drink some juice, dilute it with water, and then EAT something!

A mixture of whole-grain complex carbohydrates and protein usually works best, which is all the more reason to stick to your dietary regimen. The main purpose of the diet for hypoglycemia is to prevent drops in glucose, NOT to fix them after the fact.
—*Dr. Lorna Walker*

Q. Recently, I got stuck in New York-New Jersey traffic on the way to my grandson's wedding. I had no way to get a quick juice or milk as we could not even exit to a rest stop! How do you deal with these unpredictable situations?

A. In order to avoid the situation you had in traffic, you must be prepared. Always carry something with you in case of emergency. An easy choice is nuts, cheese, whole wheat crackers and peanut butter. You can also carry glucose tablets; however, I prefer a food snack. Every time I leave my house, I make sure to put a snack into my purse. In addition, I stash a bag of nuts in the storage area of my car. That little baggie is always there in case I forget to bring a fresh snack. Develop the habit of taking water and that snack with you when you know you'll be away from home for more than a quick trip.

Naturally, eating throughout the day, like grazing on three meals and two snacks, will also help avoid a fall in blood sugar. For a great list of allowable snacks that you can download for free, check out Connie Bennett's website at www.sugarshock.com.
—*Roberta Ruggiero*

Hypoglycemia and Relevance to Other Medical Conditions

Q. My son (18) has prostate cancer and was treated with chemotherapy. Now he has symptoms of hypoglycemia. Is there any connection?

A. Not necessarily. With the reference to the chemotherapy being the causative agent of the hypoglycemia, it would be extremely important to know which chemotherapy was used. Symptoms of hypoglycemia can occur that are not necessarily connected to the therapy given. Further, it would be important to determine if this is truly hypoglycemia or general immune suppression related to the chemotherapy.
—*Dr. Herbert Pardell*

Q. I have hypoglycemia and hypothyroidism. Is this common?

A. The determination of commonality is very difficult because symptoms of both of these diseases seem to cross over and can be exhibited in either hypoglycemia or hypothyroidism. Decreased thyroid function will affect glucose metabolism and, in fact, will affect every part of the metabolic system, causing symptoms such as fatigue, sweating, weight gain, etc.

Hypoglycemia can give you similar symptoms. At this time, I don't know of any studies that give an exact percentage of how many people have both entities. However, again, the symptomology of these diseases can be seen in either one.
—*Dr. Herbert Pardell*

Q. I have hypoglycemia and chronic fatigue syndrome. Even though I'm on a strict hypoglycemia diet, I still can't seem to feel better. Is there anything I can do to speed the healing process?

A. Although you have not elucidated what you are doing at this time, I would assume that, under the circumstances, you are following protocols that include both diseases. The use of multiple antioxidants (which should of course include lipoic acid, selenium and chromium along with a strict diet) would help in this endeavor. Other parts of the protocol include a good exercise program along with proper rest. Each person is an individual, and the rate of healing depends on the general state of health and cannot be generalized for any one person.
—*Dr. Herbert Pardell*

Q. Even though I am on a hypoglycemia diet, I still am having a problem with candida. Can you help explain how I can control this yeast overgrowth?

A. Candida overgrowth simply represents a disturbance in the normal balance of the entities that we live with every day. There is a certain amount of bacteria, fungus, yeast, viruses and other varmints that normally coexist quietly both on and inside everyone. When this balance is disturbed (like killing off a bunch of bacteria with antibiotics), we develop an overgrowth of one or more of the surviving organisms. Normally the body will reestablish the balance but sometimes requires some assistance.

We can help this process by consuming "good bacteria" such as Lactobacillus species before, during and after exposure to antibiotics. Monistat vaginal suppositories are now available over the counter and will help to prevent the vaginitis common with antibiotic usage as well as treat an infection when it occurs. Diflucan 150 mg is a prescription antifungal that is effective in reducing the amount of yeast present and may be taken several times as necessary for management of severe yeast infections. All medications have potential side effects, so the advice and counsel of your physician is important in dealing with these problems.

Unfortunately, people who are susceptible to yeast infections seem to develop them more easily than others. I'm not exactly sure why.
—*Dr. Douglas M. Baird*

Q. I have celiac (sprue) and intolerance to gluten. I was later told I had functional hypoglycemia. Can celiac disease cause hypoglycemia?

A. Celiac disease or sprue is an intolerance to the gluten contained in grains like wheat, rye, oats, and barley. When gluten is eaten, the lining of the intestine is injured and diarrhea, abdominal pain and inability to absorb nutrients results. Celiac disease can result in hypoglycemia when nutrients (including calories) are not absorbed. This is not functional hypoglycemia, but hypoglycemia resulting from untreated celiac disease. Fortunately, if the diet for celiac disease is strictly adhered to, the hypoglycemia should resolve. Having said that, it is important to note that one can have sprue, adhere to the diet, and still have functional hypoglycemia from a diet high in sugars and refined carbohydrates. If that is the case, then you would have to adhere to a diet that avoided all sources of gluten as well as sugars and refined carbohydrates.
—*Dr. Lorna Walker*

Q. My girlfriend has been diagnosed with natal hypoglycemia. From what I can make of the information available, low blood sugar can be caused by pregnancy and/or childbirth. Do you have any information on this condition?

A. Glucose mismanagement disorders are common to pregnancy. Both gestational diabetes and gestational hypoglycemia can occur. Many times the condition disappears after giving birth, but sometimes the stress of pregnancy is suspected of bringing out a condition that the woman is prone to anyway. In either case, the diet for hypoglycemia is compatible with pregnancy, as it is a healthy one. Be sure to have your girlfriend check with her doctor.
—*Dr Lorna Walker*

Q. I was curious about a link between hypoglycemia and migraine headaches. For example, can hypoglycemia be a trigger for migraines or migraine-like headaches?

A. Some patients with hypoglycemia experience headaches when their blood sugar drops. However, there is no direct correlation between migraine headaches and hypoglycemia. Migraine triggers are dietary, hormonal, psychological, and physiological (such as lack of sleep). These can also be triggers for hypoglycemia. Before determining if there is a correlation in your case, it is imperative that you get your hypoglycemia under control. Check our website for dietary advice. A diet diary is imperative if you want to determine what triggers your headaches and/or hypoglycemia. —*Dr. Lorna Walker*

HYPOGLYCEMIA AND SUPPLEMENTS

Q. I am hypoglycemic. I've heard and read that I should take chromium picolinate. How does it help, and how much should I take?

A. Chromium, whether it is given as chelate, picolinate or polynicotinate, helps insulin work better to transport glucose to the cells. A big problem with insulin resistance is a deficiency of chromium and other trace elements. Without a mineral analysis, it is safe to take chromium as picolinate or chelate or polynicotinate at 200 to 400 mcg per day for adults. If you had a mineral analysis, we might recommend higher amounts.

One word of caution: if you have high insulin levels and all your insulin is not sensitive, the chromium may initially activate it and you could experience worse blood sugar symptoms. If that happens, reduce or eliminate the chromium until you get further testing to see what you need.
—*Jay Foster*

Q. I am hypoglycemic and have been taking an herbal supplement from the local health food store that has St. John's Wort and Ma Huang in it. Are there any health risks with this combination?

A. The Ma Huang may be dangerous. Many people using it report cardiac stress symptoms, including rapid heartbeat. The FDA is trying to get it banned. St. John's Wort is okay, but 50 mg. (morning and night) of 5-HTP is better, although you cannot take either if you are on an SSRI drug such as Paxil, Prozac or Zoloft.
—*Jay Foster*

Q. My nine-year-old daughter was diagnosed as having hypoglycemia. I changed her diet, which consisted of a large amount of sugar and fruit juices. She was doing quite well until I started giving her a vitamin/ mineral supplement. I thought this was a good idea. Why does she seem worse since I added this chewable?

A. I just addressed this problem in a recent article that I wrote in the *Journal of Longevity*. Your child may be allergic to some of the additives in the supplement. Our research has shown that about seven percent of the population has chemical sensitivities to a variety of things like synthetic food colors, food dyes, binders, and fillers. (Incidentally, many food dyes, binders, and emulsifiers have been linked to attention deficit hyperactivity disorder [ADHD] and hyperactivity alone.) For example, although kids prefer chewable vitamin supplements, all chewables contain the exact same chemicals, which we know promote hyperactivity. Unfortunately, there's no known technology for creating a chewable without using these chemicals. For those kids who are chemically sensitive, hypoallergenic nutritional supplements are the answer.

—*Dr. Stephen J. Schoenthaler*

HYPOGLYCEMIA AND SUGAR/SUGAR SUBSTITUTES

Q. If my blood sugar dips too low and I am not near food, can I take GLUCOSE tablets?

A. Taking glucose tablets will raise your blood glucose but only briefly. It will drop again very quickly. The best way to control hypoglycemia is to avoid a drop in blood sugar. Instead of carrying around glucose tablets, try keeping emergency snacks with you at all times. Nuts are very portable as are whole grain crackers with peanut butter or cheese. They can be carried easily in your purse or briefcase.

—*Dr. Lorna Walker*

Q. I've eliminated Aspartame and NutraSweet. Can I have Splenda?

A. Research shows that the artificial sweetener Splenda, also known as sucralose, is a chlorinated sucrose derivative. I do not recommend it. For more information, look it up on the internet. What you might try is Stevia. Stevia comes from a South American tree. It is natural, comes in pills, powder and liquid. I do not find the taste great, but other people find it very appealing. Also, research shows that it will do no harm.

—*Dr. Nancy Appleton*

Q. How much sugar can a hypoglycemic ingest safely in one day?

A. I think a hypoglycemic should ingest very little sugar. This includes all forms of simple sugar such as sucrose, glucose, fructose, maltose, dextrose, honey, barley, malt, maple syrup, rice syrup, brown sugar, raw sugar, turbinado sugar, corn sweetener, corn syrup solids, liquid cane sugar, concentrated fruit juice, and fruit juice. The less, the better.

There is plenty left to eat. If you eat fruit, eat it with protein and fat to control your blood sugar level. The fruits that have the least amount of sugar are melons and berries.

—*Dr. Nancy Appleton*

Q. I have read that you should eat sugar to stabilize your glucose levels. But this makes me feel worse and out of control. I have been diagnosed with hypoglycemia. I don't understand why this is suggested so often. Any suggestions?

A. There is a possibility you may be reading advice for diabetics who are going into insulin shock. When this happens, they need to "jolt" their sugar levels up with a candy bar, orange juice or straight sugar. This is **NOT** advisable for people who are hypoglycemic.

Sugar is a big NO for you and must be avoided! Go back and read everything you can on hypoglycemia. Borrow books and CDs from your local library, especially the ones I recommend in the appendix of this book, and browse the internet. Some sites have a list of allowable foods for people with hypoglycemia, a daily blog and even suggestions for online support groups.

Also reread the sections in this book about diet and recommended foods and menus.

Be sure you are not reading advice for people with diabetes! Remember, the low blood sugar in hypoglycemia is the pancreas's response to eating sugar and refined carbohydrates. Low blood sugar connected to diabetes is completely different from that connected to just hypoglycemia.
—*Roberta Ruggiero*

HYPOGLYCEMIA AND PRESCRIPTION DRUG TREATMENT
Q. What kind of medicine do you take for hypoglycemia? I've had it for 10 years, but nothing has ever been done about it.

A. Unfortunately, many of us feel that a "pill" will alleviate our symptoms or pain, but with hypoglycemia, only a change in dietary habits can produce results. So the answer to your question is NO...there is no medication for hypoglycemia. Diet, stress and lifestyle changes are usually necessary. Most often eliminating offending foods like white sugar, white flour, alcohol, caffeine and tobacco make a huge improvement in your health. It is unfortunate you didn't seek help and had to suffer for ten years! I can't stress enough that EDUCATION is crucial if you are faced with any condition or disease! Please read as much as you can about hypoglycemia. The more you know, the better you will be able to handle and control your symptoms.
—*Roberta Ruggiero*

Q. Do you have a list of physicians who treat reactive hypoglycemia with glucagon (also known as GlucaGen)? I had one glucagon shot years ago when I was first diagnosed and I felt wonderful. However, all physicians since told me that is wrong as I am only borderline diabetic.

A. Sorry, but I can't agree with treating hypoglycemia with glucagon. It is one of the opposing hormones of insulin (i.e. has the opposite action of insulin), but treating reactive hypoglycemia with it doesn't solve the problem. **Reactive** hypoglycemia means the pancreas reacts to rapid elevations of blood glucose by secreting too much insulin. This is caused by eating a diet high in refined carbohydrates and sugars. Your pancreas was not designed to handle these constant "highs," so it begins secreting too much insulin. Thus what it is doing you have taught it to do by eating the Standard American Diet (SAD!). The answer is to change your diet. The pancreas gets a rest and you get healthier!
—*Dr. Lorna Walker*

Q. I was recently diagnosed with hypoglycemia. My doctor prescribed a drug that has proved, in many cases, to reduce all signs of hypoglycemia. The drug is called Proglycem. Do you have any available information on this drug?

A. Proglycem (also known as Hyperstat) is a powerful drug used in the treatment of hypertensive emergency and "pathologic hypoglycemia due to insulinoma." An insulinoma is a tumor of the insulin-secreting cells of the pancreas. Functional hypoglycemia is not listed as one of the clinical indications for administration of this drug. In functional hypoglycemia, the insulin-secreting cells over secrete insulin in response to eating sugar and/or excessive refined carbohydrates. That is one reason why the fasting glucose levels in functional (reactive) hypoglycemia are usually within normal range. It is also why the condition is best treated with diet and lifestyle changes. I would surely consult a reputable endocrinologist before taking Proglycem for this condition.
—*Dr. Lorna Walker*

Q. I have hypoglycemia and usually can keep my symptoms under control. However, they flared up when I was given prednisone for a rash. Does this medication usually cause adverse reactions if one has low blood sugar?

A. Prednisone will many times put diabetes out of control, so one may expect that it could do something similar in a hypoglycemic. One has to

The Do's and Don'ts of Hypoglycemia   Roberta Ruggiero

weigh the possible benefit against any detriment in prescribing almost any medication. Many times, these reactions are difficult or impossible to predict. Just make sure that your doctor is reminded of this reaction should a cortisone product ever be necessary in the future.

—*Dr. Douglas M. Baird*

Q. Are there any studies showing that birth control pills can cause some women to suffer from hypoglycemia?

A. As most women can attest, hormones can affect blood sugar levels. Just prior to getting their period, many women crave sugar. However, this is not true reactive hypoglycemia.

The short answer to your question is: no, birth control pills do not cause reactive hypoglycemia. Poor diet and lifestyle, coupled with a genetic predisposition, do. If you already have hypoglycemia, birth control pills might make it more difficult to control. However, some women with large fluctuations in hormone levels have been helped by the pill.

—*Dr. Lorna Walker*

HYPOGLYCEMIA AND EXERCISE

Q. I have hypoglycemia. I understand the importance of exercise. However, when I do exercise, even just walking, I feel very dizzy and short winded. Is this a symptom of hypoglycemia and just normal?

A. Stop your exercise until you see your healthcare professional. Dizziness is a symptom of hypoglycemia but should not come about as a result of exercise unless you are exercising during a low blood sugar attack. Moreover, dizziness combined with feeling short winded or out of breath, warrants a physical exam and tests to eliminate the possibility of any serious ailment or condition.

—*Roberta Ruggiero*

HYPOGLYCEMIA AND HYPNOSIS

Q. Is hypnosis recommended for hypoglycemia? I'm having a very difficult time with my diet. I can't seem to break my caffeine habits. I'm willing to try this, but would this be the easy way out?

A. Although you could use hypnosis to try to gain control over longstanding habits, it is not necessarily the best treatment choice. The essential issue here is controlling cravings. The cravings you have are biologically driven.

You may think they are a matter of will or psychological in some way, but when your blood sugar drops, you have little control over your food choices. Therefore, if you are following a proper hypoglycemic diet, the "cravings" should dissolve away. There are some food habits that are emotionally based. You will be able to see these once you have cut away the biologically driven ones. Examples include eating comfort foods when upset or bored, or having a "relationship" with food in the place of the relationship you yearn for. If you feel you are eating from emotional need, a brief course of individual psychotherapy is a better treatment choice.

Regarding coffee, you must remember that caffeine is a drug from which you must withdraw slowly. Go slowly and replace it with a healthy alternative. Don't overlook how powerful this morning ritual is, and brew herbal/green tea instead of coffee if that is your replacement.
—*Dr. Nancy Scheinman*

HYPOGLYCEMIA AND SUPPORT GROUPS

Q. I'm 19 years old and have hypoglycemia. I was about 17 when they finally figured out what was wrong with me. I want to be a voice for hypoglycemia, but I don't know where to start. I would love to become more involved with the Hypoglycemia Support Foundation. I don't feel enough people know about this. If there is a way I can help, please let me know.

A. Your question and others like it bring me to tears. It is important that those of us with hypoglycemia help spread the word—hypoglycemia is real and not a fad disease or condition!

Here is how you or anyone else can help spread the word about hypoglycemia and/or the HSF:

◀ **Learn everything you can and then SHARE it. Start with family and friends, then your school, doctors, hospitals and the media. Tell those closest to you about hypoglycemia, your personal story and that you would like everyone to know about this condition because it could be playing a role in many of their lives without them even knowing it.**

◀ **If you are in school, especially high school and college, consider doing a term paper on hypoglycemia.**

◀ **Contact your local media (newspapers/magazines) and ask them to write about this condition, or write an article yourself and submit it.**

◀ Contact your local radio and TV stations, and ask them to do a show on teenagers and hypoglycemia and tell them the reason why. That should spark their interest. You can also speak at your local schools and hospitals. This would be easier to arrange if you had a physician or nurse behind your efforts. See if you can get a healthcare professional to assist you with your goals, which, by the way, are commendable!

—*Roberta Ruggiero*

Q. Are there any support groups for hypoglycemia?

A. Support for people with hypoglycemia is growing, but support groups are not as common as for other conditions or diseases. Check your local newspapers, magazines, hospitals for a list of support groups and/or classes in your area.

Some support groups may not be specifically for hypoglycemia, but you may find they work for you. Other groups, such as those focused on eating a low-carb diet or stress reduction, could be very beneficial as well and are usually are attended by health-conscious individuals. Try stress-relief classes, exercise or yoga classes, nutrition classes and even cooking classes. All of these would help anyone suffering from low blood sugar problems.

Consider joining Food Addicts in Recovery Anonymous (FA), www. foodaddicts.org, which is an international fellowship of men and woman who have experienced difficulties in life as a result of the way they eat. Members join FA either because they could not control their eating or because they were obsessed with food. FA's program of recovery is based on the Twelve Steps and Twelve Traditions of Alcoholics Anonymous. They make use of AA principles to gain freedom from addictive eating. There are no dues, fees or weigh-ins at FA meetings. Membership is open to anyone who wants help with food. Check their website for a chapter in your area.

You can also form your own support group. Two, three or four people gathered together, sharing and offering hope, can be the best medicine any doctor could prescribe. Put a small ad in your local paper or in a health-food store saying, for example, "Seeking Others with Hypoglycemia for Support and Encouragement." As the number of members grows, ask a local doctor, nurse or nutritionist to help lead and guide the group. Also, check out the organizations and books listed in the Appendices of this book for discussion topics and ideas. Good luck!

—*Roberta Ruggiero*

66 *I have had a lot of success quitting drinking by changing my diet—every symptom that I suffered corresponded with hypoglycemia and everything that cured it as well—I just received surgery for severe gastrointestinal disorders and the doctor kept telling me that there's no such thing as hypoglycemia—I was crying in the doctor's office from all my confusion.*99

—**Rosa**

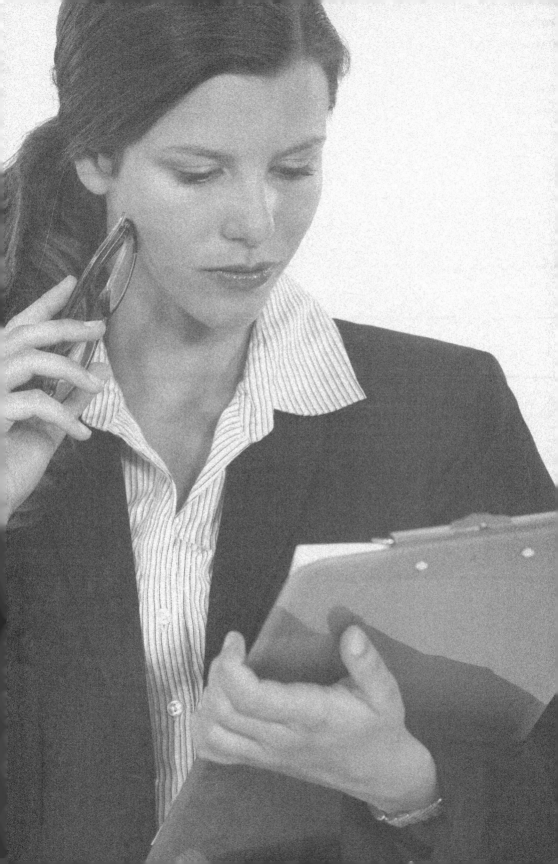

“ *My 12 year old daughter was diagnosed about six months ago with hypoglycemia. The doctor was great but only gave us a sheet of diet suggestions, not really enough for long-term success. While discussing my frustration to a few new acquaintances, one of the mothers understood my feeling – her son was diagnosed over a year ago. She proceeded to tell me about your book, especially the chapter on Children with Hypoglycemia and how much it helped her and her family. I ordered a copy, received it and read it in a day. Thank you so much, it was just what my daughter and our family needed!* ”

—Theresa

Chapter 6
Survey Results

WITNESSING MIRACLES

I was never so excited to write a chapter in my book as I am at this very moment. When I wrote the first edition, my only desire was to share with you my personal experiences, plus what I learned from trial and error, on how to control and live with hypoglycemia. Never did I imagine my path would take me to where I am today—witnessing miracles on a daily basis!

If any of you have visited the HSF's website and Facebook page during 2015–2016, you would have realized that after almost 4 years of monthly blogs, I suddenly stopped posting. Even my daily sharing of vital information pertaining to everything helpful to someone with low blood sugar, came to a slow crawl.

Why so?

My husband was diagnosed with a very rare and severe form of leukemia—large glandular lymphocyte leukemia (LGL). For ten years, he fought with all his might to keep up with his day-to-day rituals, even though he was in and out of hospitals. At times, I didn't think he would make it home. But he did. Then 2 years ago, his condition took a turn for the worse. In one year, he was hospitalized twice, in a nursing home, in rehab, on 3 months of antibiotics, and even 3 months of hyperbaric oxygen therapy. Blood transfusions, which had worked in the past, couldn't save him at the end. After 4 weeks in hospice, he lost his brave battle and passed away on Oct. 24, 2016.

I mention this scenario because it was the darkest time of my life. I was not only physically exhausted, I was emotionally drained. Seeing the love of my life slipping away and not being able to help or save him cut to my heart and soul! However, in between this gloom and doom period, rays of sunshine were starting to tiptoe in. I didn't quite see it but I felt it!

It started with a phone call in January 2016 from Wolfram Alderson, then Executive Director of the Institute for Responsible Nutrition, based in San Francisco . I was introduced to Wolfram by Connie Bennett, author of Sugar Shock, who was putting on a Sugar World Summit and wanted us to be involved. Although that summit was delayed, Wolfram, his colleague, Leslie Lee, and I started putting our ideas together about how we could join the "eliminate sugar revolution." Very slowly, and despite my time and energy being at an all-time low, our working and friendship relations blossomed. When I causally mentioned I would like to repeat the hypoglycemia questionnaire from 1989, both Wolfram and Leslie eagerly said, "Let's do it!" Consequently, they were responsible for taking our past Hypoglycemia Questionnaire to another level. They re-evaluated, designed and implemented a new version…more medical and technical. Today, I am so proud, honored and excited to share with you the results of that survey!

HYPOGLYCEMIA SURVEY

Background

The Hypoglycemia Support Foundation, Inc. and the Institute for Responsible Nutrition conducted an online survey targeting individuals who experience hypoglycemia. The purpose of this survey was to characterize their experiences and diagnostic processes, and to observe connections between reactive hypoglycemia and type 2 diabetes. Further, the survey's aim in the collection of these data is to legitimize the condition within the medical community.

The survey remains open for responses. If you would like to participate, you can access it by visiting www.hypoglycemia.org and clicking on "Take our Hypoglycemia Questionnaire.

Summary of Results

At the time of this edition, 1161 responses have been collected. Those who took the survey are primarily adults (95%), and more than 97% believe they have experienced hypoglycemia. Interestingly, 63% of all respondents report they know they have experienced hypoglycemia; however, only 47% report their condition had been diagnosed by a physician and only 29% have had hypoglycemia confirmed by an oral glucose tolerance test (OGTT).

The most commonly reported symptoms of hypoglycemia include:

- Fatigue (82%)
- Shakiness (79%)
- Dizziness (70%)
- Mood swings (64%)
- Confusion (62%)
- Nervousness (58%)
- Hunger (58%)
- Headaches (55%)

- Heart palpitations (51%)
- Cravings for sweets (50%)
- Cold hands and feet (47%)
- Food cravings (46%)
- Blurred vision (43%)
- Depression (42%)
- Outbursts of temper (40%)
- Insomnia (32%)
- Crying (30%)
- Loss of consciousness (15%)*

  Loss of consciousness is an indicator of severe hypoglycemia with neurologic impairment.

Symptoms of hypoglycemia are experienced with the following frequency:

- At least once a day (30%)
- At least once a week (30%)
- Once or twice a month (18%)
- Only occasionally (14%)

The most commonly reported triggers of hypoglycemia include:

- Skipping meals (76%)
- Stress (57%)
- Certain foods or beverages (49%)
  - Pastries or doughnuts (43%)
  - Candy (41%)
  - Desserts (39%)
  - Sweetened beverages (34%)

- Caffeinated beverages (32%)
- Alcohol (30%)
- Breakfast cereals (29%)
- Juice or smoothies (29%)
- Bread (28%)
- Pasta (27%)
- Processed snack foods, such as chips, crackers or bars (26%)
- White rice (21%)
- Starchy vegetables (14%)
- Diet beverages (11.4%)
- Sauces, spreads, dressings, or condiments (10%)
- Whole grains (6%)

- Exercise (36%)
- Illness (23%)
- Travel (13%)
- Medications (11.1%)
- Not sure (22%)

Respondents reported how they *treat* hypoglycemia once it occurs.

- Eat something with protein (41%)
- Eat slow carbs, like nuts, seeds, or whole grains (30%)
- Eat something sweet like candy or dessert (29%)
- Eat any type of food, no matter what it is (27%)
- Drink juice (23%)
- Rest (22%)
- Take glucose tablets (13%)
- Eat crackers (13%)

- Eat 15 grams of fast-acting carbohydrate, rest for 15 minutes, then check blood glucose and repeat if necessary (12%)
- Drink soda (11%)
- Administer glucagon (2%)

Our respondents reported the following steps they take to *prevent* hypoglycemia episodes from occurring.

- Eat frequently (61%)
- Eat balanced meals and snacks containing protein, fat, fiber and carbohydrate (57%)
- Avoid trigger foods (49%)
- Follow a consistent routine with eating, medications, exercise, work, sleep (37%)
- Eat before being physically active (32%)
- Regularly measure blood glucose with a glucose meter (34%)
- Proactively measure blood glucose (10%)
- Only measure glucose when hypoglycemia suspected (24%)
- No steps taken to prevent hypoglycemia (14%)

Prevention helped reduce frequency or severity of symptoms or both in 67% of respondents.

Diabetes

Other blood glucose- or insulin-related diagnoses:

- Pre-diabetes (10%)
- Insulin hyper-secretion (7%)
- Type 2 diabetes (3%)
- Type 1 diabetes (< 1%)
- Previously had type 2 diabetes or pre-diabetes, but no longer do (3%)

Of those diagnosed with type 2 diabetes or pre-diabetes (n=179), 68% experienced hypoglycemia prior to their diagnosis, 12% did not experience hypoglycemia prior to their diagnosis, and 20% weren't sure or couldn't remember.

Of those who reported they suffered from hypoglycemia prior to a diagnosis of type 2 diabetes or pre-diabetes (n=120), 100 indicated they suffered with low blood sugar from 2 months to 60 years. It was not possible from the responses to determine and average length of time before diagnosis, however, the distribution is as follows:

- < 6 months: 9
- 6 months - 2 years: 6
- 2-4 years: 4
- 5-9 years: 10
- 10-14 years: 13
- 15-19 years: 6
- 20+ years: 27

Additional responses indicated the following for lengths of time suffering before a diagnosis of type 2 diabetes:

- "years": 12
- "entire life": 5
- "since childhood": 4
- "since I was a teen": 2
- "for decades": 2

Most of the above responses clearly indicate prolonged periods of time. The most ambiguous response is "years." By definition, "years" must mean two or more years. Combining all responses together then, 85% (of those who specified a duration) experienced hypoglycemia for two or more years prior to a diagnosis of diabetes.

Of those who went on to be diagnosed with type 2 diabetes or pre-diabetes, 45% were not told that hypoglycemia could be a risk factor for diabetes compared with 43% who were advised of the relationship.

To rule out medication-induced hypoglycemia, we asked if respondents were taking any of 19 glucose-lowering medications currently available – 94% reported they were not taking any of those medications. Glucophage (Metformin) was the most commonly taken medication within the group at the low rate of less than 3%. Only 1% of respondents takes insulin.

Alarmingly, 25% of those taking our survey who have been diagnosed with diabetes or pre-diabetes report they will intentionally let their blood glucose run high to prevent hypoglycemia.

The Patient Experience

Only 40% of respondents indicated they understand hypoglycemia well enough to satisfactorily manage their symptoms. It is impressive that this rate is as high as it is considering only 17 percent believe hypoglycemia is well understood by their health care team and only 23 percent report their concerns about hypoglycemia are taken seriously by their health care team.

By contrast, respondents were nearly twice as likely to indicate their loved ones understand hypoglycemia well (35%) and take their concerns seriously (54%). If loved ones can see these individuals are suffering, why can't clinicians?

Discussion

Often, when hypoglycemia is discussed in the medical and research communities, it is often described as the unintended consequences of insulin use by those with diabetes. However, our respondents overwhelmingly reported they experience hypoglycemia (97%), are non-diabetic (86%), and are not taking any glucose-lowering medications (94%). It is our hope that this finding and our other survey results will underscore that hypoglycemia does indeed occur in the general population, not just in those who are controlling their diabetes with medication.

There is little published about how reactive hypoglycemia can precede diabetes and perhaps even serve as a warning sign that the disease is developing. Among our respondents with type 2 diabetes, a majority (68%) experienced hypoglycemia before their diabetes diagnosis. Of those individuals, 85% experienced hypoglycemia for 2 or more years before being diagnosed with diabetes. Had they understood that hypoglycemia is a warning sign of developing diabetes and had they known what to do about it, they might have potentially intervened to prevent the disease or delay its onset, thus potentially improving their quality and length of life.

We believe the phenomenon of reactive hypoglycemia is increasing in the general population because of the easy availability of overly-processed food, abundant in refined flour and sugar, which delivers excessively large amounts of rapidly absorbed glucose and fructose (both types of sugar).

Large amounts of rapidly absorbed glucose leads to an excessive rise in blood glucose followed by an excessive rise in insulin. That relatively high level of insulin then works too well, lowering blood glucose too low resulting in reactive hypoglycemia. With frequent spikes, insulin levels increase even further over time contributing to insulin resistance and eventually, type 2 diabetes.

The rise of blood glucose and insulin after a meal is completely normal. What's abnormal, relatively speaking, is our food. Processing of food removes the fiber in whole foods that naturally protects us from large, rapid glucose spikes.

Fructose does not directly affect blood glucose. However, it is still implicated in this process. Fructose is metabolized exclusively by the liver. When it is absorbed in large amounts, which happens when one consumes free sugar (added sugar or sugar freed from fiber in whole foods, such as in juice), the liver is overwhelmed and converts fructose to fat. That fat is either exported in the blood in the forms of cholesterol and triglycerides, or it is deposited in the liver. A fatty liver becomes an insulin resistant liver, which further contributes to the development of diabetes.

Martinez Steele et al published in the *BMJ Open* (2016) that a majority of Americans' calories (58%) are delivered in the form of ultra-processed foods, and those ultra-processed foods deliver 90 percent of our added sugar intake.[1] Our food is evolving more quickly than our genes. Our metabolism cannot keep up with the amount of bioavailable glucose and fructose we ingest from processed foods.

We suggest reactive hypoglycemia is evidence of metabolic dysfunction induced by processed foods that, if left unaddressed, could result in type 2 diabetes. *Reactive hypoglycemia should be considered a call-to-action for the prevention of type 2 diabetes and other advanced forms of metabolic disease.*

HEALTH CARE OPPORTUNITIES

Our survey identified that educational opportunities exist for both those who suffer from hypoglycemia as well as their care teams. Most of our respondents reported they have low confidence in their health care team's knowledge of hypoglycemia (83%), and their health care team does not take their concerns about hypoglycemia seriously (65%). Many respondents indicated they feel unsupported and even ostracized by the medical community. Real responses include:

"Doctors are not educated and are no help. You are left alone."

"I don't go to the doctor for this anymore. They have no clue."

"I have suffered with hypoglycemia since I was a child. When I discuss my symptoms with my doctors, I am always told that there is no such thing as hypoglycemia. I have been told my symptoms are anxiety symptoms. It is frustrating because my symptoms disappear if I eat or drink something. They disappear within 15 minutes. I think it's sad that general practitioners and endocrinologists have not taken my concerns seriously. In the past, I have monitored my glucose levels and saw that my symptoms coincided with glucose levels in the 50s and 60s. Again, my doctors told me that those numbers don't qualify as being low."

"My primary care physician doesn't think I need to take an [oral glucose tolerance test] and dismisses my concern because my blood sugar is within "normal range" when I've been tested in the office."

"My son is 12 years old and has had terrible temper problems and learning disabilities from about 4 years old until now. I have had his thyroid, hormones, allergies and vitamin levels checked and all were normal. I told our doctor that I thought he had hypoglycemia and she brushed it off as "hangry." Well, Hangry has put dozens of holes in our walls, broken doors and broken toys. Hangry doesn't recognize any feelings of hunger until it's too late. The more we push him to eat, at that point, the more he insists that he isn't hungry and the spiral gets worse. I have been to so many different specialists and no one mentions food or hypoglycemia. I figured it out myself and I'm so thankful I did. When he eats, every 2-3 hours and has a variety of proteins and vegetables, he is a different person."

"The healthcare professionals I have seen since I was diagnosed with hypoglycemia 17 years ago have always treated me like they thought it was a joke. As a result, I am still battling it with only help from loved ones."

Considering most respondents feel alone and unsupported in their management of hypoglycemia, it is no surprise that 60% report they experience hypoglycemia as often as once a week or more. The same percentage also admit they do not know how to satisfactorily manage their symptoms. It is apparent from these responses that patients won't improve until clinicians improve.

Improving patient outcomes and experience should be simple, so long as clinicians are trained to interpret reactive hypoglycemia as a red flag for type 2 diabetes. Better educated clinicians can empower patients to not just treat hypoglycemia as it occurs, but to prevent it, regain their quality of life, and prevent diabetes from developing at the same time.

One area that could easily be improved is diagnosis. Hypoglycemia is difficult to diagnose because it is impractical for a person experiencing hypoglycemia to get to a lab for a blood draw when symptomatic, glucose meters are known to be imprecise in the low range, epinephrine can kick in and raise blood glucose between the time hypoglycemia is experienced and blood glucose is measured, and oral glucose tolerance tests are often too short to observe reactive hypoglycemia. Alternatively, a patient could be so nervous for the OGTT that cortisol could elevate their blood glucose preventing hypoglycemia during the test.

Despite being challenging, diagnosis should still be pursued. Only 41% of respondents indicated they underwent an oral glucose tolerance test, the gold standard in diagnosing reactive hypoglycemia. We recommend a 3-hour (at least) OGTT that includes measurement of insulin (to observe for hyperinsulinemia). Primary care physicians can diagnose reactive hypoglycemia. A referral to a specialist is not necessary.

If an oral glucose tolerance test does not confirm hypoglycemia, but symptoms are consistent with reactive hypoglycemia, a physician might consider recommending a trial of a low-carbohydrate, minimally processed diet. It is a relatively easy, low-cost, low-risk intervention. If a patient's symptoms improve, isn't that most important? If they don't improve, then reactive hypoglycemia can be ruled out.

Our intention is to increase the percentage of patients who are properly diagnosed with hypoglycemia by a physician, informed that hypoglycemia could be a sign that diabetes is developing, and equipped with practical ways of both successfully managing hypoglycemia and preventing the onset of diabetes.

EDUCATIONAL OPPORTUNITIES

So, what should an intervention to both manage reactive hypoglycemia and prevent diabetes look like?

Severe hypoglycemia is an emergency necessitating immediate action. The quickest way to correct it, if the person is conscious, is to consume refined flour or sugar, because the glucose in each is rapidly absorbed. Flour- and sugar-rich foods are readily available so this makes for a convenient solution. Glucose tablets, for example, are an alternative, but they are far less available than food. Many of our respondents indicate they turn to flour- or sugar-rich foods to treat hypoglycemia.

We believe focusing on treatment alone without any ongoing preventive measures is short-sighted. It may correct the emergency at hand, but it only adds fuel to the cycle of metabolic dysfunction that the patient is experiencing. It's trading hypoglycemia now for diabetes later.

A better way is to focus on preventing hypoglycemia altogether, while educating on ways to treat hypoglycemia thoughtfully, rather than reactively. The tenets of this education are:

- Test finger stick blood glucose to identify trends
- Identify personalized triggers of hypoglycemia
- Eliminate those triggers
- Eat a source of slow-absorbing carbohydrate, such as nuts, when blood glucose is borderline low or mild symptoms are present, but it is not yet an emergency
- Treat hypoglycemia when it occurs in the manner that the American Diabetes Association recommends: 15 grams of fast-acting carbohydrate, followed by 15 minutes of rest, then checking blood glucose and repeating if necessary
- Prepare for these last two points by preemptively carrying sources of slow-absorbing carbohydrate and fast-absorbing carbohydrate, at least until hypoglycemia becomes an uncommon event

Dietary triggers of reactive hypoglycemia among our respondents include starches, sweets, sweet beverages, caffeinated beverages, alcohol, and surprisingly, diet beverages. If one were to eliminate or greatly reduce starches, sweets, and alcohol in their diet to prevent reactive hypoglycemia, this would certainly help to prevent type 2 diabetes as well. Type 2 diabetes is an intolerance to starches and sugars, and excessive alcohol makes the liver fatty and insulin resistant just as fructose does.

While caffeine is a big offender for hypoglycemia, we don't have reason to believe at this point that caffeine contributes to diabetes. However, it's worth mentioning that many caffeinated beverages are also sweetened, so an intentional reduction in caffeine could result in consuming fewer sweeteners, which certainly could help to prevent diabetes.

The fact that greater than 11% of respondents indicated that diet beverages trigger hypoglycemia is worth discussing since these beverages deliver no calories, glucose or fructose and are assumed to exert no metabolic effects. Could it be that simply the taste of sweetness induces metabolic dysfunction?

Epidemiological evidence suggests that consumption of non-nutritive sweeteners (NNS), mainly diet sodas, is associated with increased risk of developing obesity, metabolic syndrome, and type 2 diabetes[2,3]. Pepino describes in *Physiology and Behavior* that theories exist to explain how NNS might promote metabolic dysregulation, namely that

- Non-nutritive sweeteners interfere with glucose control through learned responses

- Non-nutritive sweeteners trigger insulin secretion through their sweet taste, and

- Non-nutritive sweeteners disrupt gut microbiota which leads to metabolic dysregulation.[4]

The experience of our respondents seems to corroborate that NNS may not be as metabolically inert as once believed. More research is clearly needed in this area.

Some additional surprising foods traditionally touted as "healthy" were also reported as triggers of hypoglycemia. These include starchy vegetables (14%) and whole grains (6%). This finding supports the need for a personalized approach to eliminating trigger foods. One person's safe food may be another's trigger. Patients will need guidance on how to observe their diet, blood glucose values, and symptoms to identify precisely what their dietary triggers are.

ADDITIONAL OPPORTUNITIES

Treating Hypoglycemia

It's noteworthy that eating protein was the most commonly indicated form of treatment for hypoglycemia (41%) among our respondents. This is surprising since protein slows gastric emptying (compared to carbohydrate) and is only converted to glucose by way of gluconeogenesis after digestion and absorption. It seems like a slow and indirect way to raise blood glucose in an emergency. *Perhaps respondents are confusing advice to eat protein at all meals and snacks to prevent hypoglycemia with what they should do to treat hypoglycemia.*

Only 12% of respondents treat hypoglycemia the way the American Diabetes Association (ADA) recommends. Perhaps too few are informed of the guideline or they find it impractical. When it's apparent that blood glucose is low and one needs to eat, perhaps it's unlikely that a person would take the time to identify precisely 15 to 20 grams of fast-acting carbohydrate. It seems more likely they would just examine their environment and eat the most accessible food (or beverage) that they think has the best chance of raising their blood glucose. They may also feel too confused or hungry to limit their intake to only 15 to 20 grams. Additionally, there are likely many people who wouldn't see the need to check their blood glucose after eating, as the ADA recommends, if they were already feeling better.

Steps can be taken to increase the practice of the ADA's treatment guideline, including educating patients on why it's important and what 15 to 20 grams of fast-acting carbohydrate looks like. We can encourage patients to always carry 15 to 20 grams of fast-acting carbohydrate with them and help them identify foods that are portable and provide the recommended dose. We can convince them this is important to thoughtfully treat hypoglycemia, rather than having to be responsible for responding to their own emergency while it's happening. Planning in advance will also ensure they have the right amount of food to improve their condition without over-treating it and causing yet another episode of reactive hypoglycemia later.

Real Food

We recommend avoiding processed foods, since processed foods induce the metabolic dysfunction contributing to reactive hypoglycemia and type 2 diabetes. Instead, we encourage a real food, or whole food, diet. Real food contains fiber, which protects us from excessive amounts of glucose and fructose.

One major objection to real food is that it requires preparation and cooking. Indeed, home cooking is probably the best way of controlling the quality and healthfulness of your diet. We recognize that many people were not taught to cook or have abandoned their skills for convenience foods, diverting more of their time toward other priorities. As a society, we need to overhaul our food culture. We need to embrace cooking at home once again, family meal times, and prioritizing quality food, because we won't change the trajectory of diet-induced disease until we do so.

Clinicians can help by prescribing real food, cooking, shopping at farmers' markets, and even gardening. However, our communities also need cooking classes, access to affordable high-quality food, and programs to support these.

Time Between Meals

Many respondents (76%) report that skipping meals triggers hypoglycemia and 61% practice eating frequently to keep their blood glucose elevated enough. If dietary triggers of reactive hypoglycemia were removed, perhaps the practice of eating frequently wouldn't even be necessary. Perhaps without the insult of trigger foods, insulin levels would normalize, hypoglycemia could be avoided, and one could fast for more than three to four hours without incidence, as our bodies are designed to do. Eating less frequently would help with insulin sensitivity, which could also help to prevent the later development of diabetes.

Eating less frequently is inadvisable for those who experience frequent episodes of hypoglycemia, but increasing time between meals could be a long-term goal once dietary triggers are removed, blood glucose is more stable, and frequent episodes subside.

Managing Hypoglycemia in the Setting of Type 2 Diabetes

Among those with diabetes, more than 25% indicated they intentionally let their blood glucose run high to prevent hypoglycemia. This action is another example of a short-term trade-off with long-term consequences. These individuals need help in getting reactive hypoglycemia under control so they can successfully manage (or perhaps even reverse) diabetes. A real food, low-carbohydrate, high-healthy fat diet could accomplish both goals simultaneously.

It's also important to avoid dismissing a patient's concerns about hypoglycemia because their hemoglobin A1c is non-worrisome. Hemoglobin A1c is an average of blood glucose control. It's certainly possible that extreme highs and extreme lows can produce a normal average value. That doesn't mean that what the patient is experiencing is benign.

Beyond Food

Hypoglycemia educational needs extend beyond nutrition. Education should address self-care practices, such as stress management, keeping a consistent schedule, how to travel safely, precautions to take when ill, and how to exercise safely. Further, individuals experiencing hypoglycemia should be encouraged to become more self-aware and notice how their habits affect their condition. Lastly, becoming part of a supportive community focused on eating healthy, real food can be extremely helpful to sustain well-being. The Suppers Programs, based in Princeton, New Jersey, provides an excellent model for doing this – however, there are many organizations around the world that can provide similar support - you just have to look for them.

REFERENCES

1. Martínez Steele E, Baraldi LG, Louzada MLDC, et al Ultra-processed foods and added sugars in the US diet: evidence from a nationally representative cross-sectional study *BMJ Open* 2016;6:e009892.

2. Brown RJ, de Banate MA, Rother KI. Artificial sweeteners: a systematic review of metabolic effects in youth. *Int J Pediatr Obes*. 2010;5(4):305–12.

3. Swithers SE, Martin AA, Davidson TL. High-intensity sweeteners and energy balance. *Physiol Behav*. 2010;100(1):55–62.

4. Pepino MY. METABOLIC effects of non-nutritive sweeteners. *Physiol Behav*. 2015;152(0 0):450-455.

5. The Suppers Programs: http://www.thesuppersprograms.org/

"Low blood sugar comes up at just about all of our meetings. Whether it's people in recovery, or emotional eaters or carboholics, or diabetics, or people with leaky guts, or insomniacs, just about everybody who comes to our program is dealing with hypoglycemia. Probably the largest single chunk of our facilitator training is about recognizing low blood sugar and understanding how so many different symptoms and diagnoses are driven by it. It also features large in the programs I teach at The College of New Jersey. It's crazy to me that we train counselors and social workers with no food education or nutrition and then we end up diagnosing them with mental health issues."

—**Dorothy Mullen, Founder of The Suppers Programs**

What does our survey mean for you? Some takeaways.

So, you read the results. Now, where does that leave you? Whether you've conquered and controlled all your symptoms, slowly recovering one day at a time, or still stuck in limbo – I am sure you're asking, "How do the results apply to me? What can I take away from all these percentages and statistics?"

As you read the survey results above, I'm sure you could relate with many if not all of them, or you know someone who can. One thing you can certainly take away from the survey results is that you are not alone! Hypoglycemia is real and you have a lot of company. As we continue to bring awareness to this disease and work to get the medical community on board, you can also take away the fact that work is being done to educate both the public and the medical community about hypoglycemia.

You also can share the results with your friends, family, and care team and encourage anyone you know who also experiences hypoglycemia to take the survey, which is accessible on the HSF website – www.hypoglycemia.org

That said, here are some things you can do for you – right now:

1) **Learn as much as you can about hypoglycemia**. Read every book you can get your hands on that discusses the subject. One may contradict another; others will be confusing and difficult to understand. Nevertheless, you will learn something from each of them. Remember, too, you don't have to read everything all at once. You can read a chapter, a page or a few paragraphs at a time. Learning takes time, energy, patience, and commitment. Don't give up. Just do it gradually and consistently. Don't say you don't have the time or ability–you do! I cannot stress enough that knowledge and understanding of the causes, effects and treatment of this condition are imperative now.

2) **Keep a symptom diary**. This is a daily account of everything you eat for one week to ten days. In one column, list every bit of food, drink and medication you take and at what time. In the second column, list your symptoms and the time at which you experience them. Very often you will see a correlation between what you have consumed and your symptoms.

3) **Make a list of your symptoms** and bring it to a healthcare professional along with your diet/symptom diary and the questions and concerns

generated from all your reading on hypoglycemia. There is no substitute for a medical diagnosis and treatment plan!

4) **Visit our website**s – www.hypoglycemia.org and www.hypoglycemiaKIDS.org. Can't find a physician? Want to know if you need the glucose tolerance test? Questioning what you should eat? Wondering if you will become diabetic? Worried that your two-year-old might have hypoglycemia? Your questions may seem endless, and it is impossible to answer all of them individually. But the good news is that many of your concerns may be addressed on our website. Visit it today! You will find pages of up-to-date information on hypoglycemia and personal stories that will inspire and uplift you. And don't miss out on almost four years of HSF blogs…a wealth of timeless information you can't afford to miss!

5) **Visit us on Facebook** and join the conversation. www.facebook.com/HypoglycemiaSupport Here you will discover up close and personal news and views on every aspect of hypoglycemia. The best part is that you will meet a family of others brave enough to share their personal stories. Perhaps you will see yourself in some of their experiences. More importantly, you might find a suggestion or two that work for you or have a suggestion that will help others. We all have knowledge to share!

6) **Most important!** Read and re-read the above results of our Hypoglycemia Questionnaire. The information sheds a rare glimpse into this "most confusing, complicated, misunderstood and misdiagnosed condition." A special thank you to Dietitian/Nutritionist, Leslie Lee for evaluating the results and giving us an easy to understand assessment of a complicated condition. If any one area concerns you, go back through the pages of this book, our website and Facebook pages to hopefully find your answers. Remember, that nothing ever takes the place of a medical diagnosis and treatment plan! Seek help, reach out and form a group of individuals who will be your personal advocates!

YOU must take the first step. Education, preparation and commitment are key to recovery. Believe in you, believe in miracles!

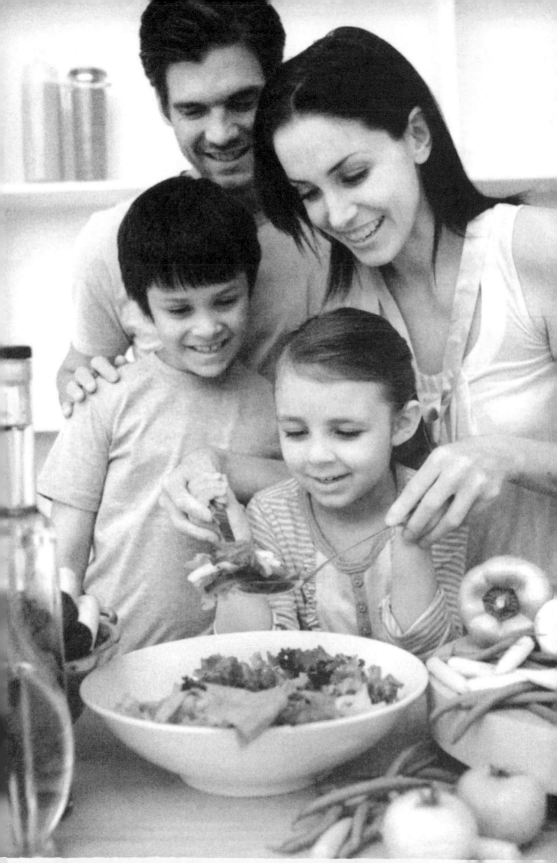

" *The amount of residual alcohol in a savory dish depends on the temperature and time. Typically wine or other acidic liquids are used to deglaze a pan in preparation for making a sauce. This is high heat and the alcohol burns off rapidly to the point that there is little discernible left. In a dish where wine is added early in the cooking process, the alcohol is gone before the dish is finished and adds flavor but not booze. In the case where the wine is added to a relatively low heat dish just prior to serving, there is alcohol content but normally there is not enough on a percentage basis to make much difference to a hypoglycemic patient. It sort of depends on how rigid one wants to be with dietary restriction. The short answer is that it probably doesn't make much difference.* "

—Dr. Douglas M. Baird

Chapter 7
Recommended Foods & Menus

SMORGASBORD OF DIETARY DELIGHTS

From Robert's Favorite Italian Recipes to Her Everyday, Simple Diet Suggestions

I often get e-mails from hypoglycemics having a difficult time with knowing what to eat. Some feel there's nothing they can have that is enjoyable anymore. Others feel totally deprived. When I realized I had the opportunity to revise my book again, I knew instantly that I had to add more recipes to this section. Those suffering from hypoglycemia need to know that there are plenty of choices and that the food, whether a meal or a snack, can be delicious and easy to prepare.

Since food is both a necessity and a token of love and affection, I thought I would start by sharing some favorite recipes that I've cooked for family and friends over the years. I invited my niece, Lisa, and her son, Anthony Piscazzi, to contribute their favorites also. Anthony is a culinary chef, graduated from the famous Le Cordon Bleu in North Miami, Florida. His passion for cooking encompasses style, presentation and taste. Anthony challenges himself by creating old-fashioned Italian recipes with an innovative flair while preparing one-of-a-kind dishes that he's excited to share with family and friends…and with you, my readers.

But before we move on to the recipes, I want to pass along some interesting information gleaned from conversations with my nephew, Anthony. I was anxious to find out if the public is changing their eating habits. So I asked him the following question: Are your customers more health conscious today when they order any of your specialties? Anthony was quick to reply, "Not everyone is, but more than average. I am now asked to go easy on the cheese or to broil that piece of meat or fish instead of frying it — or they want to know if they can have a side of vegetables instead of pasta. And when ordering a salad, most want their dressing on the side so they can control calories." I finally had to ask the big one….Do they skip dessert? He responded, "Not really, but they share." Let's hope that's because they are conscious of calories and sugar content…not just the extra cost!

And now that I've provided a little insight into my family's favorite pastime — eating and cooking — and the evolution of eating habits in the U.S., I am sharing some simple suggestions that make my food preparation and cooking as easy and effortless as possible. Being prepared and stress free are the secrets to success.

Following are recipes and simple cooking suggestions, then a list of recommended snacks and finally a list of foods that hypoglycemics need to avoid and those that are permissible.

So as the saying goes…Bon appétit!

"I can't believe how much better I feel after going on a hypoglycemia diet. There is no way I am going back to my old eating habits…it is not worth the pain!"

ESCAROLE AND BEANS

2-3 heads of escarole, cleaned and cut up

4 tbsp. of olive oil

5 cloves of garlic

1 large can of navy beans

1 pound of sweet or hot sausage

Heat oil in a large pot, then brown garlic and sausage thoroughly and sauté. Add escarole, then chicken broth and stir well. Bring to a boil, lower heat, add navy beans and simmer for 45 minutes. Add salt and pepper to taste. Serve with grated cheese.

ZUPPA LENTICCHIE (LENTIL SOUP)

1 pound lentils

2 large carrots cut bite size

1 medium onion

2 garlic cloves

2 stalks of celery cut bite size

2-3 fresh tomatoes cut small

8 cups of water

Rinse lentils, place in a soup pot, cover with 8 cups of water. Let come to a boil. In a separate pan, sauté garlic, onion, celery, carrots and fresh tomatoes. Salt and pepper to taste. Cook about 20 minutes and then add to lentils. Simmer together 45 minutes or until lentils are tender. You can add more water if needed.

EGGPLANT CARBONARA

2 large eggplants

½ cup of olive oil

1 large chopped onion

1 cup of crushed tomatoes

2 celery stalks diced

½ cup of green or black olives, pitted and diced in small pieces

¼ cup of wine vinegar

Salt/pepper to taste

Cut eggplant into cubes and fry in olive oil. When browned, remove eggplant from pan. In same oil, sauté onion and celery until tender. Return eggplant back to pan. Add tomatoes, olives, wine vinegar, sugar, salt and pepper. Simmer 20 minutes, stirring frequently.

POACHED SALMON

4 4-oz. salmon fillets

2 cups chicken stock

1 bunch fresh dill tied

½ lemon squeeze

1 tbsp. butter

Place salmon in chicken stock, bring to a boil and reduce heat to low. Place dill, lemon juice and butter in the pot/pan. Cover and cook till fish is easily flaked with fork…approx. 7 minutes.

LEMON CHICKEN OVER BROWN RICE

1 cup brown rice

1 2/3 cup of water

½ cup of olive oil

4 tbsp. butter

2 cloves garlic

1 tbsp. shallots

¾ cup white wine

2 ½ tsp. lemon juice

1 ½ pounds chicken, cut into 6-oz. fillets

¼ cup chopped fresh parsley

1 ½ cups chicken stock

2 tsp. of oregano

¼ cup chopped fresh basil

Combine the brown rice and water in a small sauce pan. Bring to a boil, reduce heat to low and cook until all the water is absorbed (about 25 minutes). Add olive oil in a skillet over medium heat, add chicken fillets, and cook for 2 to 4 minutes. Then turn, add garlic and shallots, reduce heat to medium low, adding white wine, fresh lemon juice, chicken stock, butter, parsley, oregano and fresh basil, cooking until chicken reaches 165 degrees. Season with salt and pepper to taste. Serve hot over brown rice.

BAKED TILAPIA

2 lbs. Tilapia

2 green peppers sliced

2 red peppers sliced

1 onion sliced

1 lemon sliced

5 garlic cloves

2 tsp. butter

¼ cup olive oil

Pre-heat oven to 325 degrees. Place tilapia in a baking pan. Rub with butter and season with salt and pepper to taste. Top each with a slice of lemon, onion, red and green peppers and garlic cloves. Cover baking dish with foil and bake 25 to 30 minutes, until vegetables are tender and the fish flakes.

ROASTED PEPPER SALAD

1 large jar of roasted peppers ▶ or you can roast your own by placing 5-6 peppers in the oven and bake or broil until skin is blackened. Then place in brown bag and allow to cool. The skin will peel right off, allowing you to slice them lengthwise in $^1/_4$ inch to $^1/_2$ inch pieces.

1 can black olives

1 jar artichoke hearts

1 can chickpeas

3 cloves garlic

¼ cup fresh basil

Olive oil...just drizzle lightly

Sea salt and pepper

Small mozzarella balls (bocconcini) are optional

Drain the roasted peppers and slice them very thin (1/4 inch). Place in a large bowl and add the drained olives, chickpeas and artichoke hearts. Then add the garlic, basil, olive oil. Salt and pepper to taste. Serve cold.

SHRIMP PRIMAVERA

3 tomatoes peeled and chopped

1/2 cup water

¼ cup onion chopped

2 tsp. snipped fresh basil

1 lb. fresh shrimp

1/3 cup Parmesan cheese

1 cup mushrooms, sliced

1/3 cup tomato paste

¼ cup parsley

Salt and pepper to taste

2 garlic cloves, minced

1 lb. fresh asparagus

2 cups of brown rice

In medium sauce pan combine tomatoes, mushrooms, water, tomato paste, onion, parsley, basil, salt, pepper and garlic. Boil gently, uncovered, 20 minutes, stirring occasionally. Add shrimp. Heat approximately 7 minutes until shrimp is orange or cooked.

Meanwhile cook asparagus in a small amount of water, covered, for 3 minutes and drain. Cook rice. Arrange asparagus and shrimp mixture over rice on plate. Sprinkle Parmesan cheese.

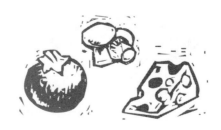

4 hardboiled eggs, peeled and cut in half

½ lb. Boar's Head salami (can even add prosciutto)

½ lb. Asiago or provolone cheese

1 can olives

1 jar of fresh roasted peppers

1 flat can anchovies

1 large jar or 2 little jars artichoke hearts

Homemade (see above recipe) or store-bought carbonara, at least 16 oz.

½ lb. shrimp...cold, peeled and deveined

Any marinated vegetables

Arrange lettuce leaves on a large platter, and place the meats and cheese on the leaves. Keep them on one side of the plate. On the other side, place the cut, hardboiled eggs and drained shrimp. Put the peppers and the artichoke hearts in a small bowl and mix well. Put the carbonara and any marinated vegetables in separate bowls. The anchovies and olives can be placed as you wish. I place salt, pepper and olive oil on the table in case anyone wants added flavor or spices.

Serve with whole wheat breadsticks, rice crackers, and millet bread. If you are symptom free and want to eat a piece of Italian bread, keep it small.

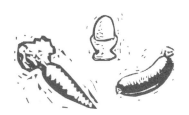

Roberta Ruggiero

The Do's and Don'ts of Hypoglycemia

BAKED FISH A LA SALSA

Fish filets (tilapia, trout or snapper)

1 green pepper chopped

1 large onion chopped

1 stalk of celery chopped

1 can diced tomatoes

1 small can mushrooms

Pinch of salt

¼ tsp. cayenne pepper

SAUTÉ green pepper, onion, celery until soft. Add mushrooms, canned tomatoes, salt, pepper. Mix all together. Place on top of fish filets. Bake at 325 degrees for approx. 15 minutes (depends on the thickness of the fish). If you like more spice, add a dash of Tabasco.

BROILED SALMON WITH DILL SAUCE

Salmon filets

¼ cup low calorie sour cream

¼ cup light mayonnaise

1 cucumber sliced thin

1 stalk fresh dill chopped (can use dried dill)

1 tbsp. sweet relish

PLACE salmon on baking pan. Mix other ingredients together. Brush the top of the fish with oil, then broil and serve with sauce on the side or cover the fish with the sauce, then bake or broil.

CANNED WILD SALMON SALAD

1 15 oz. can of wild pink or red salmon

1-2 tsp. chopped onions

1/2 cup chopped celery

2 Tbsp. mayonnaise

1 tsp. yellow prepared mustard

1 Tbsp. sweet pickle relish

PREPARE a green salad with washed and chopped lettuce, adding slivers of raw vegetables. Then make the salmon dish. Drain the liquid from the salmon and place it into a bowl. Do not remove the bones and skin from the fish. These contain valuable nutrients and they will disappear into the mixture. Add the other ingredients to the salmon, stir gently, and it's done.

Toss the vegetable salad with a simple dressing of olive oil and arrange the salad covering a luncheon or dinner plate. In the center of the salad, serve a heaping 1/2 cup of salmon salad. On the side, include a slice of whole grain bread with olive oil or butter and you have an easy, nutrient rich lunch or dinner.

SHRIMP NEW ORLEANS

1 lb. shrimp

1 green and 1 sweet red pepper, chopped

1 large onion, chopped

1 large can whole peeled tomatoes

1 bay leaf

Pinch of salt

1/8 tsp. cayenne pepper

SAUTÉ peppers and onions until soft. Then add canned tomatoes, shrimp, bay leaf, pinch of salt and cayenne pepper. Cook until shrimp is no longer translucent. Serve over jasmine rice.

TURKEY MEAT LOAF ITALIAN STYLE

1lb. ground turkey

1 cup shredded mozzarella cheese

3/4 - 1 cup chopped onion

1/3 cup chopped parsley

1 cup rolled oats

2 Tbsp. tomato paste

1 lightly beaten egg

3 cloves of chopped garlic

1 Tbsp. dried Italian herb mixture (you can use purchased "Italian Herbs" or make your own mixture from dried oregano, rosemary, thyme, etc.)

1/2 teaspoon salt

1/4 tsp. ground black pepper

COMBINE all ingredients in a large bowl while your oven preheats to 350 degrees. Then place the mixture into an oiled baking dish. A loaf pan or glass baking dish works well. Loosely cover the meat mixture with a piece of aluminum foil so the cheese does not burn during baking. Cook approximately one hour. You can tell when it's done when the loaf pulls away from the sides of the baking dish. Let cool for at least 15 minutes before serving.

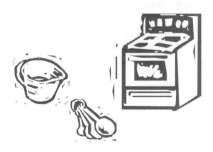

1 lb. veal cut into small pieces

½ chopped onion

1 large bell pepper cut in thin slices

½ tbsp. chopped parsley

3 cloves of chopped garlic

¼ cup fresh basil

½ cup olive oil...enough to cover pan

1 large can crushed tomatoes

1 cup of red wine

Salt and black pepper to taste

SAUTÉ the veal and turn occasionally until lightly browned. Then add garlic, onion, parsley, tomatoes and wine, and simmer for about 20 minutes. Then add the peppers and cook another 10 to 15 minutes or until veal is tender to the touch. Sprinkle the basil on top before serving on brown rice or whole wheat pasta.

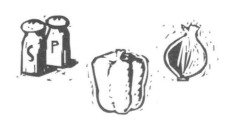

SIMPLE COOKING SUGGESTIONS

- I always cook two chickens...one to eat the night I cook and the other to save for leftovers. I cut up the chicken for chicken salad, chicken stir fry or chicken and vegetable wraps.

- I combine yellow and green squash, red peppers and onions. Bake them with just a little black pepper and sea salt, and then drizzle some olive oil on top. Bake in oven until tender. This can be used with any broiled or baked chicken, fish or lean meats.

- For fish, I love fillet of sole, flounder, cod and salmon...and serve it two to three times a week for dinner. I always make extra so I can have it for lunch the next day.

- Green vegetables are big in my house...escarole, romaine lettuce, arugula, fennel, cabbage, artichokes, broccoli, spinach, string beans, zucchini, Brussels sprouts...all fresh and just steamed or baked.

- I always have hardboiled eggs in the refrigerator.

- I usually serve an entree with side vegetables and brown rice, couscous or half sweet potato.

- Although I prefer fresh/homemade chicken salad, I do use canned chicken breast (in water) occasionally. Drain and flake, then add onions or scallions, celery, black pepper and very little mayo.

- I make an extra-large London broil, slice it very thin and serve it for dinner. (I marinate it in garlic, olive oil, soy sauce and black pepper.) I use the leftovers the next day and wrap the London broil slices over steamed asparagus as a snack.

- To spice up any vegetable, simply sauté olive oil with some garlic cloves and dribble over steamed vegetables...cauliflower, broccoli, peas, mushrooms, zucchini.

- Egg omelets...I love them and they are so easy to make. For 2-4 servings, use two eggs and two additional egg whites. Beat the egg mixture well and add any set of ingredients...eggs with broccoli and cheese, eggs with peppers and onions, eggs with mushroom and ground red pepper flakes. The possibilities are endless. Finish with sea salt and pepper to taste.

- There are other whole grains besides whole wheat, barley and oats. Give bulgur, millet, and quinoa a try.

- Be creative with spices. My favorites are ground black pepper, crushed red pepper, garlic, basil, parsley, oregano, paprika and cinnamon. Try cumin, curry, sage, thyme, caraway and rosemary.

- Use beans (pinto, kidney, lentils) whenever you can. They provide an excellent source of protein, complex carbohydrates, fiber, vitamins and minerals. A dish with beans, whole grains and a bit of protein is an economical way to maintain health and a steady blood sugar.

- Take advantage of the internet. There are recipes that you can download for free, and many sites are perfect for someone with hypoglycemia or just health-conscious individuals. Start by visiting the following: www.healinggourmet.com, www.wholefoodsmarket.com, www.jamieoliver.com, www.atkins.com, www.SouthBeachDiet.com, www.cookinglight.com and www.eatingwell.com.

- I highly suggest you visit Connie Bennett's website at www.sugarshock.com. Connie has an incredible list of allowable foods that you can download for free—a must to have at your fingertips!

- NOTE: There are stages of hypoglycemia. Some foods can be eaten when your blood sugar is under control, some sparingly when you have a few symptoms, and some foods must be avoided completely when your symptoms are out of control. It is at this time that a diet/symptom diary can be your best friend!

SUGGESTED HEALTHY SNACKS

- Cottage cheese on whole wheat crackers
- Hardboiled egg
- Greek yogurt (sugar free) with crushed almonds, some fresh raspberries or strawberries
- Nuts (almonds, cashews, pecans, walnuts) with apple slices
- Celery sticks stuffed with cashew or almond butter
- Sliced tomato and mozzarella
- Small tomato stuffed with tuna, chicken, egg or shrimp salad
- Shrimp cocktail
- Hummus on cucumber or pepper slices
- Grilled eggplant slices with ricotta cheese…served warm or hot
- Grilled Portobello mushroom topped with a slice of mozzarella cheese
- Turkey and cheese slices wrapped in lettuce
- Slices of avocado and tomato on whole wheat bread
- Carbonara on rice crackers
- Marinated roasted peppers with anchovies or sardines on brown rice crackers
- Sliced turkey breast rolled around string cheese…can add a slice of tomato
- Any leftover meat, fish or vegetables from the previous night's supper. A small piece of chicken, slice of turkey or steak. Add a slice of tomato or a few asparagus, string beans or broccoli florets and you have a great mid-morning or afternoon snack. Control portion size. This is a snack, not a meal.

RECOMMENDED FOODS

NOTE: The following list of recommended foods and menus is just a guideline. You must remember that everyone's body chemistry is different. Therefore, adjustments must be made to meet individual needs. Size of portions depends on weight and symptoms. READ the section on INDIVIDUALIZING YOUR DIET before incorporating the menus into your diet program.

MEATS: All kinds of fresh, preferably organic meats.

POULTRY: Without skin—chicken, turkey, Cornish hens, duck, pheasant.

FISH: Flounder, turbot, sole, halibut, grouper, cod, haddock, salmon, red snapper, scallops, tuna, shrimp, lobster, crab.

DAIRY: Whole milk, skim milk, cheeses (farmer, cottage, ricotta, mozzarella), eggs, butter and yogurt.

GRAINS: 100 percent whole wheat bread, brown rice, millet, oatmeal, buckwheat, oats, whole wheat pasta and rice noodles.

NUTS & Seeds: Almonds, cashews, walnuts, pecans, chestnuts, sunflower seeds, pumpkin seeds.

VEGETABLES: Artichokes, asparagus, avocado, beans, beets, broccoli, Brussels sprouts, cabbage, carrots, cauliflower, celery, chives, collard greens, corn, cucumber, eggplant, endive, garlic, kale, lettuce, mushrooms, mustard greens, okra, onion, parsley, peas, peppers, potatoes, pumpkin, radish, rhubarb, spinach, sprouts, tomatoes, zucchini, and yams.

BEVERAGES: Water, vegetable juice, herbal tea, seltzer, clear broth. Occasionally, decaffeinated coffee or weak tea.

FRUITS: Avocado, strawberries, apples, peaches, pears, oranges, watermelon, tangerines, berries, plums, grapefruit, honeydew.

FOODS TO AVOID

DESSERTS: Anything containing white sugar, such as, candy, cakes, pastries, custard, jello, ice cream, sherbet, pudding, cookies, breakfast cereals, and commercially baked breads. Avoid honey and other forms of sugar, such as brown, raw, and turbinado.

GRAINS: Anything containing white flour, such as packaged breakfast cereals, gravies, white rice, refined corn meal, white spaghetti, macaroni, noodles and refined bakery goods.

MEATS: Lunch meats, bacon, sausage, processed meats (most contain corn sugar), meat or meat products with artificial colors, flavorings or preservatives.

BEVERAGES: Alcohol, caffeine, all sugared soft drinks, and fruit juices.

FRUITS: Dried fruits (figs, dates, raisins). Fruit juices can be tolerated at times if diluted. Avoid EXCESSIVE amounts of fresh fruit.

Artificial Sweeteners like NutraSweet, Equal, Spoonful and Saccharine.

Note: Tobacco should be avoided entirely.

Bacon and sausage are permitted if organic with no preservatives, additives, MSG or nitrates.

> *"What, do I have to give up my sugar and now my coffee? You've got to be kidding! What's my alternative? There has to be one.!"* —Rick 2010

66 *I have been a hypoglycemic since I was 4!*
I am only 13 now but I thought I would have
to live with this disease forever but now I
know that if I eat right and stay right I will
maybe not even have to keep a small
chocolate bar in my back pocket anymore! 99

—**Kyleigh**

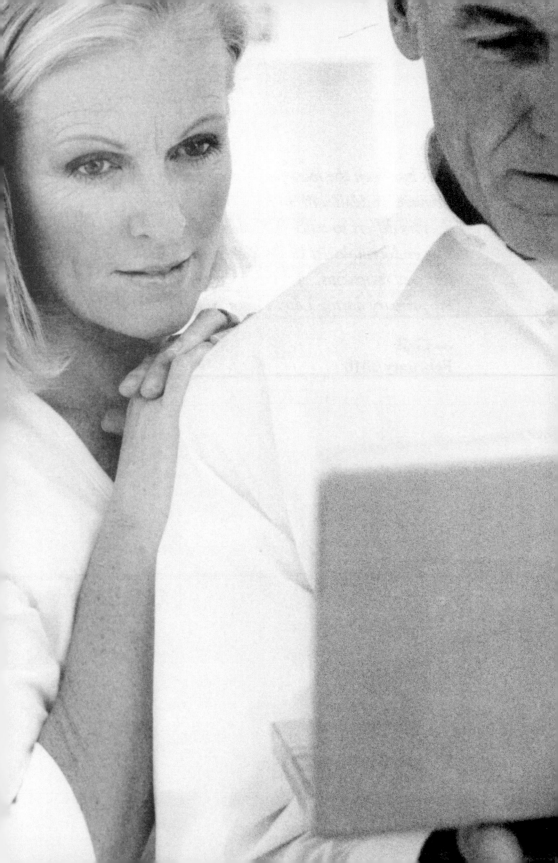

66 *This has been the most frustrating health issue I have ever dealt with so far. The opinion of doctors differs so much it's really unbelievable. The endocrinologist laughed at me and said the test was ridiculous...yet I was diagnosed by my primary doctor. I don't know what to do!* 99

—**Gail**

Chapter **8**
Want to Help the HSF?

REACHING FOR THE STARS...

On January 24, 2010, I received the following e-mail from Gwen Cooper.

> *"WOW–I've had hypoglycemia for over 25 years, in control for over 15 years until recently. Finding your site has been wonderful-I didn't know you existed. I would like to talk to you personally about what we do and how we could work together. Please visit www.florida.healthcharities. org. I will contact you this week-Can't wait to connect!"*

I was excited and eager to talk to Gwen and see what she had in mind. I must admit though, I was very skeptical. The HSF has had many offers of help over the past 30 plus years, but too often the "opportunity" placed before us turned out to be what we could do for "them" instead of what they could do for the HSF.

Not so this time. Gwen Cooper is President and CEO of Community Health Charities of Florida, a federation of Florida's top health charities, and she wanted the HSF to be a part of CHC!! She actually wanted to raise money for us, at no cost to us! Her dreams and goals for the HSF are the same as ours, and she immediately got started by talking with me about how to get involved with CHC. Within about six months, the HSF was a full member of Community Health Charities of Florida, and our name was placed in front of thousands of employees throughout Florida.

In June of 2010, Gwen came to South Florida....We were finally going to meet! It was at this meeting that Gwen said..."You're the best kept secret....You must get out there for all the world to see....That's the only way you can raise the money you need to educate and help people."

Start with a gala...plan for the best and the biggest...**reach for the stars!!!!**

So here we are in September and, as this 4th edition goes to press, just a few weeks away from the HSF's first fundraising gala. It will take place at the Hyatt Regency Pier Sixty-Six in Fort Lauderdale, Florida, on October 14, 2011. We are anticipating 200 to 300 guests!

Our goal is to raise money, not only for South Floridians but also for all those worldwide who suffer from this insidious disease. With the funds, we hope to continue our advocacy and support of hypoglycemics and their loved ones through education, workshops, support groups, research projects and social media like Facebook, Twitter, e-newsletters and our brand new website, www.hypoglycemia.org.

What is great about Community Health Charities of Florida is that fundraising can take place anywhere, anytime, from any city or town in the U.S. and also throughout the world! Donations can be made through their website and/or as part of any employer's Employee Engagement Program. CHC encourages donors to designate gifts to specific charities, so when you pick the HSF or another of the wonderful charities included in CHC's portfolio, you know the money is going directly where you want it to go.

Thank you, Gwen...We couldn't have "reached for the stars" if we didn't have support from people like you. And to everyone who has made this journey possible...I am forever grateful!

For direct donations, you can always visit www.hypoglycemia.org.

*As of this printing we put on four more HSF galas. Gwen Cooper is no longer with Community Health Charities but she continues to give us her never-ending support!

HYPOGLYCEMIA QUIZ

Hypoglycemia: Do You Have It?

In the space provided below, please mark:

(1) if you have this condition **mildly**
(2) if you have this condition **moderate**
(3) if you have this condition **severe**

If you do not have the condition, leave it blank. The accuracy of this questionnaire depends upon complete honesty and serious objective thought in answering the questions. (Many of these symptoms may relate to other health problems).

1 .... Abnormal craving for sweets

2 .... Afternoon headaches

3 .... Allergies: tendency to asthma, hay fever, skin rash, etc.

4 .... Awaken after a few hours sleep/difficulty getting back to sleep

5 .... Aware of breathing heavily

6 .... Bad dreams

7 .... Blurred vision

8 .... Brown spots or bronzing of skin

9 .... "Butterfly stomach," cramps

10 .... Difficulty making decisions

11 .... Need coffee/caffeine to start morning

12 .... Unable to work under pressure

13 .... Chronic fatigue

14 .... Chronic nervous exhaustion

15 .... Convulsions

16 .... Crave candy or coffee in afternoons

17 .... Cry easily for no apparent reason

18 .... Depressed

19 .... Dizziness, giddiness or lightheadedness

20 .... Drink more than three cups of coffee or cola a day

21 .... Get hungry or feel faint unless you eat frequently

22 .... Eat when nervous

23 .... Feel faint if meal is delayed

24 .... Fatigue relieved by eating

25 .... Fearful

26 .... Get "shaky" if hungry

27 .... Hallucinations

28 .... Hand tremor (or trembles)

29 .... Heart palpitations if meals are missed or delayed

30 .... Highly emotional

31 .... Nibble between meals because of hunger

32 .... Insomnia

33 .... Inward trembling

34 .... Irritable before meals

35 .... Lack of energy

36 .... Moods of depression, "blues" or melancholy

37 .... Poor memory or ability to concentrate

38 .... Reduced initiative

39 .... Sleepy after meals

40 .... Drowsy during the day

41 .... Weakness, dizziness

42 .... Worrier, feel insecure

43 .... Symptoms of hypoglycemia appear before eating

.... **Total Score**

Add the total of all answers. A total score of less than (20) twenty is within normal limits. A higher score is evidence of probable adrenal insufficiency and/or deranged carbohydrate metabolism (hypoglycemia) and would indicate a need for further testing.

APPENDIX A

Recommended Books on Hypoglycemia

Although some of the following books date back to the late '70s and '80s, their information is "timeless" and much too important not to share.

Blood Sugar Blues, by Miryam Ehrlich Williamson, Walker & Company, New York, 2001.

Body, Mind and Sugar, by E. M. Abrahamson, M.D. and A. W. Pezet. New York, Avon Books, 1977.

Breaking The Food Seduction, by Neal Barnard, M.D., New York, St. Martin's Press, 2003.

Carlton Fredericks' New Low Blood Sugar and You, by Dr. Carlton Fredericks. New York, Perigee Books, 1985.

Dr. Atkins' New Diet Revolution, by Robert C. Atkins, M.D., New York, M. Evans, 1992.

Food, Mind and Mood, by David Sheinkin, M.D., Michael Schacter, M.D., and Richard Hutton, New York, Warner Books, Inc., 1979.

Fighting Depression, by Harvey Ross, M.D., New York, Larchmont Books, 1975.

Get the Sugar Out, by Ann Louise Gittleman, M.S., New York, Crown Trade Paperbacks, 1996.

The Hale Clinic Guide To Good Health, by Teresa Hale, London, Kyle Cathie Limited, 1996.

The Hidden Menace of Low Blood Sugar, by Clement G. Martin, New York, Arco Publishing Co., 1976.

Hypoglycemia: A Better Approach, by Paavo Airola, Ph.D., Phoenix, Health Plus Publishers, 1977.

Hypoglycemia for Dummies, by Cheryl Chow and James Chow, M.D., Hoboken, NJ, Wiley Publishing, Inc., 2007.

Hypoglycemia: The Other Disease, by Anita Flegg, Canada, The Coach Press, 2005.

Is Low Blood Sugar Making You a Nutritional Cripple? by Ruth Adams and Frank Murray, New York, Larchmont Press, 1970.

Lick The Sugar Habit, by Nancy Appleton, Ph.D., New York, Warner Books, Inc., 1986.

Low Blood Sugar Handbook, by Ed and Patricia Krimmel, Bryn Mawr, PA, Franklin Publishers, 1984.

Low Blood Sugar: Over 100 Recipes for overcoming Hypoglycemia (Recipes for Health), Martin Budd, December 12, 2013.

Low Blood Sugar: What It Is and How to Cure It, by Peter J. Steincrohn, M.D., Chicago, IL, Contemporary Books, Inc., 1972.

Nutraerobics, by Dr. Jeffrey Bland, New York, Harper and Row, 1983.

Psychodietetics, by Emanuel Cheraskin, M.D., D.M.D., William Ringsdorf, Jr., D.M.D., with Arline Brecher. New York, Bantam Books, 1978.

Seven Weeks to Sobriety: The Proven Program to Fight Alcoholism Through Nutrition, by Joan Mathews Larson, Ph. D., New York, Ballantine Publishing Group, 1997.

The Sugar Addict's Total Recovery Program, by Kathleen Des Maisons, Ph.D., New York, Ballantine Publishing Group, 2000.

Sugar and Your Health, by Ray C. Wunderlich, Jr., M.D., St. Petersburg, FL, Good Health Publications, Johnny Reed, Inc., 1982.

Sugar Blues, by William Dufty, New York, Warner Books, Inc., 1975.

Sugar Isn't Always Sweet, by Maura (Jinny) Zack and Wilbur D. Currier, M.D. Brea, CA, Uplift Books, 1983.

Sugar Shock, by Connie Bennett, C.H.H.C., with Stephen T. Sinatra, M.D., New York, The Penguin Group, 2007.

Suicide by Sugar, by Nancy Appleton, Ph.D., New York, Square One Publishers, 2009.

Cookbooks for the Hypoglycemic

The Allergy Cookbook, by Ruth R. Shattuck, New York, A Plume Book, 1984.

Cooking Naturally For Pleasure and Health, by Gail C. Watson, Davie, FL, Falkynor Books, 1983.

Atkins for Life: The Complete Carb Program for Permanent Weight Loss and Good Health, by Robert C. Atkins, M.D., New York, St. Martin's Press, 2003.

The Carbohydrate Addict's Diet, by Dr. Rachael F. Heller and Dr. Richard F. Heller, New York, The Penguin Group, 1991.

Dr. Atkins' Quick & Easy New Diet Cookbook, by Robert C. Atkins, M.D., & Veronica Atkins, New York, Simon & Schuster, 1997.

Foods For Healthy Kids, by Dr. Lendon Smith, New York, Berkeley Books, 1981.

500 Low Glycemic Index Recipes, by Dick Logue, Fair Winds Press, 2010.

The GI Diet Made Simple, by Antony Worrall Thompson with Dr. Mabel Blades & Jane Suthering, New York, Fall River Press, 2009.

Gluten Free, Wheat Free and Dairy Free Recipes, by Grace Cheetham, Sterling Publishers Company, Inc., 2009.

Glycemic Index Cook Book, by Louis Weber, Lincolnwood, IL, Publications International, Ltd., 2010.

Hypoglycemia Control Cookery, by Dorothy Revell, New York, Berkeley Books, 1973.

The Low Blood Sugar Cookbook, by Francyne Davis, New York, Bantam Books, 1985.

Dr. Lendon Smith's Diet Plan For Teenagers, by Lendon Smith, M.D., New York, McGraw-Hill, 1986.

Step-By-Step To Natural Food, by Diane Campbell, Clearwater, FL, CC Publishers, 1979.

The South Beach Diet Cookbook, by Arthur Agatston, M.D., New York, Rodale, Inc., 2004.

Sugar Free...That's Me, by Judith S. Majors, New York, Ballantine Books, 1978.

The Low Blood Sugar Cookbook, by Ed and Patricia Krimmel, Bryn Mawr, PA, Franklin Publishers, 1984.

Exercise Books for the Hypoglycemic

Aerobics, by Kenneth H. Cooper, M.D., New York, Bantam, 1972.

Aerobics For Women, by Kenneth H. Cooper, M.D., New York, Bantam Books, 1973.

The Aerobics Program For Total Well-Being, by Kenneth H. Cooper, M.D., New York, Bantam, 1983.

The Complete Book of Exercisewalking, by Gary D. Yanker, Contemporary Books, Inc., 1983.

Fit or Fat?, by Covert Bailey, Boston, Houghton Mifflin Company, 1977.

P.A.C.E.: The 12-Minute Fitness Revolution, by Al Sears, M.D., Royal Palm Beach, FL, Wellness Research & Consulting, Inc., 2010.

Stretching (30th Anniversary Edition), by Bob Anderson, Bolinas, CA: Shelter Publications, Inc., 2010.

Water Exercise, by Martha White, Champaign, IL, Human Kinetics, 1995.

Gary Yanker's Sportwalking, by Gary Yanker, New York Contemporary Books, 1987.

Yoga Made Easy, by Howard Kent, Chicago, Chicago Review Press, Inc., 1993.

Books to Help Develop a Positive Attitude

Anatomy of An Illness, by Norman Cousins, New York, W. W. Norton & Co., 1979.

The Art of Extreme Self Care, by Cheryl Richardson, New York, Hay House, Inc., 2010.

Bus 9 To Paradise, by Leo Buscaglia, New York, Fawcett, 1987.

Eat, Pray, Love, by Elizabeth Gilbert, New York, Penguin Books, 2006.

Enthusiasm Makes the Difference, by Norman Vincent Peale, New York, Fawcett, 1987.

The Gift of Change: Spiritual Guidance for a Radically New Life, by Marianne Williamson, New York, Harper Collins, 2004.

Gifts From Eykis, by Dr. Wayne Dyer, New York, Pocket Books, 1983.

Goodbye to Guilt, by Gerald G. Jampolsky, M.D., New York, Bantam Books, Inc., 1985.

The Healing Heart, by Norman Cousins, New York, Avon Books, 1983.

The Last Lecture, by Randy Pausch, New York, Hyperion, 2008.

Love, by Leo Buscaglia, New York, Fawcett Crest Books, 1972.

Loving Each Other, by Leo Buscaglia, New York, Fawcett Columbine, 1984.

Peace From Broken Pieces, by Iyanla Vanzant, New York, Hay House, Inc., 2010.

Personhood, by Leo Buscaglia, New York, Fawcett Columbine, 1978.

The Power of Now: A Guide To Spiritual Enlightenment, by Eckert Tolle, Novato, CA, New World Library, 1999.

The Power of Positive Thinking, by Norman Vincent Peale, New York, Prentice-Hall, Inc., 1952.

Pulling Your Own Strings, by Dr. Wayne Dyer, New York, Thomas Y. Crowell Co., 1978.

The Purpose Driven Life, by Rick Warren, Grand Rapids, MI, Zondervan, 2002.

A Return To Love, by Marianne Williamson, New York, Harper Collins Publishers, 1992.

The Road Less Traveled, by M. Scott Peck, M.D., New York, Simon & Schuster, 1978.

The Shack, by William Paul Young, Los Angeles, CA, Windblown Media, 2007.

The Shift, by Dr. Wayne W. Dyer, New York, Hay House, Inc., 2010.

Tough Times Never Last, But Tough People Do!, by Robert H. Schuller, New York, Bantam Books, 1983.

The Seat of the Soul by Gary Zukav, Simon & Shuster, 1990.

The Sky's The Limit, by Dr. Wayne Dyer, New York, Simon and Schuster, 1980.

Teach Only Love: The Seven Principles of Attitudinal Healing, by Gerald G. Jampolsky, M.D., New York, Bantam, 1983.

When Bad Things Happen to Good People, by Harold S. Kushner, New York, Avon Books, 1981.

Your Erroneous Zones, by Dr. Wayne Dyer, New York, Funk & Wagnalls, 1976.

Zero Limits, by Joe Vitale, Hoboken, NJ, John Wiley & Sons, Inc., 2007

Books on the Correlation Between Hypoglycemia and Learning Disabilities, Juvenile Delinquency, Mental Illness, Alcoholism and Candida Albicans

Allergies and the Hyperactive Child, by Doris J. Rapp, M.D., New York, Simon & Schuster, 1979.

Brain Allergies, by William H. Philpott, M.D., and Dwight K. Kalita, Ph.D., New Canaan, CT, 1980.

Chocolate to Morphine, by Andrew Weil, M.D., and Winifred Rosen, Boston, Houghton Mifflin, 1968.

Diet, Crime and Delinquency, by Alexander Schauss, Ph.D., Berkeley, CA, Parker House, 1981.

Eating Right To Live Sober, by L. Ann Mueller, M.D., and Katherine Ketchum, New York, NAL, 1986.

Fighting Depression, by Harvey Ross, M.D., New York, Larchmont Books, 1975.

Food, Teens and Behavior, by Barbara Reed Stitt, Ph.D., Manitowoc, WI, Natural Press, 1983.

Hypoglycemia: A Better Approach, by Paavo Airola, Ph.D., Phoenix, Health Plus Publishers, 1977.

Mind, Mood and Medicine: A Guide To The New Biopsychiatry, by Paul H. Wender, M.D., and Donald F. Klein, M.D., New York, NAL, 1982.

Psychodietetics, by E. Cheraskin, M.D., D.M.D., William Ringsdorf, Jr., D.M.D., with Arline Brecher, New York, Bantam Books, 1978.

Sugar and Your Health, by Ray C. Wunderlich, Jr., M.D., St. Petersburg, FL Good Health Publications, 1982.

The Yeast Connection, by William G. Crook, M.D., Jackson, TN, Professional Books, 1983.

The Yeast Syndrome, by John Parks Trowbridge, M.D., and Morton Walker, D.P.M., New York, Bantam, 1986.

Here is a list of organizations that supply nutritional Information and referral listings. Thank you to Connie Bennett, author of *Sugar Shock,* for contributing to this list.

The Hypoglycemia Support Foundation, Inc.
P.O. Box 451778
Sunrise, Florida 33345
www.hypoglycemia.org

AlternativeMedicine.org
1650 Tiburon Boulevard
Tiburon, CA 94920 USA
Phone (800) 515-4325
http://www.alternativemedicine.org

American Academy of Osteopathy
3500 DePauw Boulevard, Suite 1080
Indianapolis, IN 46268
Phone (317) 879-1881
http://www.academyofosteopathy.org/

American Association of Naturopathic Physicians (AANP)
3201 New Mexico Avenue, NW Suite 350
Washington, DC 20016
Phone (202) 895-1392 or (866) 538-2267 (toll free)
http://www.naturopathic.org

American Holistic Health Association

P.O. Box 17400 Anaheim, CA

Phone 714-779-6152

www.ahha.org

American Holistic Medical Association (AHMA)

12101 Menaul Blvd. Northeast, Suite C

Albuquerque, NM 87112

Phone (505) 292-7788

http://www.holisticmedicine.orgdatabase.

The Institute for Functional Medicine

4411 Pt. Fosdick Drive NW, Suite 305

P.O. Box 1697

Gig Harbor, WA 98335

Phone (800) 228-0622 Fax (253) 853-6766

www.functionalmedicine.org

International Academy of Nutrition

P.O. Box 370

Manly NSW 1655

Australia

Phone: 61(2)99770771 Fax: 61(2)99770267

Website: www.intacad.com.au

The Life Extension Foundation (LEF)

5990 N. Federal Hwy.

Fort Lauderdale, Florida 33309

Phone (954) 766-8433 or (800) 544-4440

http://www.lef.org/doctors/directoryofdoctors01.html

American Dietetic Association
120 South Riverside Plaza, Suite 2000
Chicago, Illinois 60606-6995
Phone 1 (800) 877-1600

International and American Associations of Clinical Nutritionists
(IAACN)
15280 Addison Road, Suite 130
Addison, Texas 75001
Phone (972) 407-9089
http://www.iaacn.org/http://www.eatright.org

Center for Science in the Public Interest
1220 L St. N.W.
Suite 300
Washington, D.C. 20005
Main switchboard: (202) 332-9110
Fax: (202) 265-4954

APPENDIX C

BIBLIOGRAPHY

Abrahamson, E. M., M.D., and Pezet, A. W. *Body, Mind and Sugar.* New York, Avon Books, 1977.

Adams, Ruth, and Murray, Frank. *Is Low Blood Sugar Making You a Nutritional Cripple?* New York, Larchmont Press, 1970.

Agatston, Arthur, M.D. *The South Beach Diet Cookbook.* New York, Rodale, Inc., 2004.

Airola, Paavo, Ph.D. *Hypoglycemia: A Better Approach.* Phoenix, Health Plus Publishers, 1977.

Anderson, Bob. *Stretching* (30th Anniversary Edition). Bolinas, CA: Shelter Publications, Inc., 2010.

Anderson, Linnea, M.P.H., Dibble, Marjorie V., M.S., R.D., Turkki, Pirkko R., Ph.D., R.D., Mitchell, Helen S., Ph.D., Sc.D., Rynbergen, Henderika J., M.S. *Nutrition in Health and Disease*, 17th Edition. Philadelphia, J.B. Lippincott Company.

Appleton, Nancy, Ph.D. *Lick the Sugar Habit.* New York, Warner Books, Inc. 1986.

Appleton, Nancy, Ph.D. *Suicide by Sugar.* New York, Square One Publishers, 2009.

Atkins, Robert C., M.D. *Atkins for Life: The Complete Carb Program for Permanent Weight Loss and Good Health.* New York, St. Martin's Press, 2003.

Atkins, Robert C., M.D., & Veronica Atkins. *Dr. Atkins' Quick & Easy New Diet Cookbook.* New York, Simon & Schuster, 1997.

Atkinson, Holly, M.D. *Women and Fatigue.* New York, G. P. Putnam's Sons, 1985.

Bailey, Covert. *Fit or Fat?* Boston, Houghton Mifflin Company, 1977.

Barnard, Neal, M.D. *Breaking The Food Seduction.* New York, St. Martin's Press, 2003.

Bennett, Connie, C.H.H.C., with Stephen T. Sinatra, M.D. *Sugar Shock.* New York, The Penguin Group, 2007.

Bennion, Lynn J., M.D. *Hypoglycemia: Fact or Fad?* New York, Crown Publishers, Inc. 1983.

Bland, Jeffery, Ph.D. *Your Health Under Siege*. Brattleboro, VT, The Stephen Greene Press, 1981.

Brennan, Dr. R. O. *Nutrigenetics*. New York, M. Evans and Company, 1975.

Budd, Martin L., N.D., D.O., Lic. Ac. *Low Blood Sugar*. New York, Sterling Publishing Co., Inc., 1981.

Cheetham, Grace. *Gluten Free, Wheat Free and Dairy Free Recipes*. Sterling Publishers Company, Inc., 2009.

Cheraskin, E., M.D., D.M.D., William Ringsdorf, Jr., D.M.D. and W. Clark, D.D.S., *Diet and Disease*. CT, Keats Publishing, Inc., 1986.

Cheraskin E., M.D., D.M.D., William Ringsdorf, Jr., D.M.D., with Arline Brecher. *Psychodietetics*. New York, Bantam Books, 1978.

Cheraskin, E., M.D., D.M.D., William Ringsdorf, Jr., D.M.D., and Emily L. Sisley, Ph.D. *The Vitamin C Connection*. New York, Harper & Row Publishers, Inc., 1983.

Chow, Cheryl and James Chow, M.D. *Hypoglycemia for Dummies*. Hoboken, NJ, Wiley Publishing, 2007.

Crook, William G., M.D. *The Yeast Connection*. Jackson, TN, Professional Books, 1983.

Dufty, William. *Sugar Blues*. New York, Warner Books, Inc., 1975.

Dyer, Dr. Wayne W. *The Shift*. New York, Hay House, Inc., 2010.

Flegg, Anita. *Hypoglycemia: The Other Disease*. Canada, The Coach Press, 2005.

Fredericks, Carlton, Ph.D. *Carlton Fredericks' New Low Blood Sugar and You*. New York, Perigee Books, 1985.

Fredericks, Carlton, Ph.D. *Psycho-Nutrition*. New York, Grosset & Dunlap, 1976.

Gilbert, Elizabeth. *Eat, Pray, Love*. New York, Penguin Books, 2006.

Hale, Teresa. *The Hale Clinic Guide to Good Health*. London, Kyle Cathie Limited, 1996.

Heller, Dr. Rachael F. and Dr. Richard F. Heller. *The Carbohydrate Addict's Diet*. New York, The Penguin Group, 1991.

Kent, Howard. *Yoga Made Easy*. Chicago, Chicago Review Press, Inc., 1993.

Krimmel, Patricia and Edward. *The Low Blood Sugar Handbook.* Bryn Mawr, PA, Franklin Publishers, 1984.

Logue, Dick. *500 Low Glycemic Index Recipes.* Fair Winds Press, 2010.

Lorenzani, Shirley, Ph.D. *Candida; A Twentieth Century Disease.* New Canaan, CT, Keats Publishing, Inc., 1986.

Martin, Clement G. *Low Blood Sugar: The Hidden Menace of Hypoglycemia.* New York, Arco Publishing Co., 1976.

The Merck Manual of Diagnosis and Therapy, Twelfth Edition. Rahway, NJ, Merck Sharp & Dohme Research Laboratories, Division of Merck & Co., Inc., 1972.

Milam, James R., and Katherine Ketcham, *Under the Influence*, New York, Bantam Books, 1981.

Nutrition and Mental Health. Hearing before the Select Committee on Nutrition and Human Needs of the United States Senate. Berkeley, CA, Parker House, 1977.

Page, Melvin E., D.D.S., and H. Leon Abrams, Jr. *Your Body is Your Best Doctor.* New Canaan, CT, Keats Publishing, 1972.

Passwater, Richard A. *Supernutrition.* New York, Pocket Books, 1975.

Pritikin, Nathan, with Patrick M. McGrady, Jr. *The Pritikin Program for Diet and Exercise.* New York, Grosset & Dunlap, 1979.

Rapp, Doris, J., M.D. *Allergies and the Hyperactive Child.* New York, Simon & Schuster, 1979.

Reed, Barbara. *Food, Teens and Behavior.* Manitowoc, WI, Natural Press, 1983.

Richardson, Cheryl. *The Art of Extreme Self Care.* New York, Hay House, Inc., 2010.

Ross, Harvey, M.D. *Fighting Depression.* New York, Larchmont Books, 1975.

Schauss, Alexander. *Diet, Crime and Delinquency.* Berkeley, CA, Parker House, 1981.

Sears, Al, M.D. *P.A.C.E.: The 12-Minute Fitness Revolution.* Royal Palm Beach, FL, Wellness Research & Consulting, Inc., 2010.

Saunders, Jeraldine, and Ross, Harvey, M.D. *Hypoglycemia: The Disease Your Doctor Won't Treat*, New York Pinnacle Press, 1980.

Smith, Lendon, M.D. *Feed Yourself Right*. New York, McGraw-Hill, 1983.

Smith, Lendon, M.D. *Foods For Healthy Kids*. New York, Berkeley Books, 1981.

Thompson, Antony Worrall with Dr. Mabel Blades & Jane Suthering. *The GI Diet Made Simple*. New York, Fall River Press, 2009.

Tolle, Eckert. *The Power of Now: A Guide to Spiritual Enlightenment*. Novato, CA, New World Library, 1999.

Truss, C. Orion, M.D. *The Missing Diagnosis*. Birmingham, The Missing Diagnosis, Inc., 1983.

Vanzant, Iyanla. *Peace From Broken Pieces*. New York, Hay House, Inc., 2010.

Vitale, Joe. *Zero Limits*. Hoboken, NJ, John Wiley & Sons, Inc., 2007.

Warren, Rick. *The Purpose Driven Life*. Grand Rapids, MI, Zondervan, 2002.

Weber, Louis. *Glycemic Index Cook Book*. Lincolnwood, IL, Publications International, Ltd., 2010.

Weil, Andrew, M.D., and Rosen, Winifred. *Chocolate to Morphine*. Boston, Houghton Mifflin Co., 1983.

Weller, Charles. *How To Live With Hypoglycemia*. New York, Doubleday, 1968.

White, Martha. *Water Exercise*. Champaign, IL, Human Kinetics, 1995.

Williamson, Marianne. *A Return To Love*. New York, Harper Collins Publishers, 1992.

Williamson, Marianne. *The Gift of Change: Spiritual Guidance for a Radically New Life*. New York, Harper Collins, 2004.

Wunderlich, Jr., Ray C., M.D. *Sugar and Your Health*. St Petersburg, FL, Good Health Publications, Johnny Reed, Inc., 1982.

Young, William Paul. *The Shack*. Los Angeles, CA, Windblown Media, 2007.

Yudkin, John, M.D. *Sweet and Dangerous*. New York, Bantam Books, 1972.

Zack, Maura, and Currier, Wilbur D., M.D. *Sugar Isn't Always Sweet*. Brea, CA, Uplift Books, 1983.

INDEX

121, 130, 140, 164

dizziness, 32, 34, 37, 46, 61, 93, 99, 104, 113, 121, 145, 173-174

dried fruits, 58, 134, 167

Dyer, Dr. Wayne, 79, 179-180, 186

E

electroconvulsive shock therapy (ECT), 23, 30, 37-39, 76,

exercise, 7, 23, 39, 69, 71-73, 82, 96, 113, 115, 129, 139, 145, 147, 178, 187-188

F

fainting, faintness, 28, 39, 46, 50, 52, 94-95, 104, 124-125, 174

fatigue, 34, 46, 57, 73, 94-95, 99, 101-102, 109, 113-114, 121, 138, 139, 173-174, 185

forgetfulness, 46

Foster, Jay, 41, 119, 141

Fredericks, Dr. Carlton, 47, 61, 175, 186

fructose, 58, 136, 142

functional hypoglycemia, 39, 45, 74, 120, 140, 144

G

gastric bypass, 133

gestational diabetes, 140

glucola, 61

glucose, 58, 133, 142

glucose tolerance test (GTT), 23, 28, 32, 34, 39-40, 47-48, 50, 61-63, 64, 74, 94, 98, 102, 110, 113, 120-122, 126

gluten, 140, 177, 186

glycemic index, 135, 177, 187-188

H

Harris, Dr. Seale, 48

headaches, 26, 32, 35, 37, 46, 57, 61, 92, 98-100, 113, 121, 140, 173

health & beauty, 81-90

heart palpitations, 46, 113-114, 121, 123, 174

Health Emergency Card, 50, 95

Health Recovery Center, 107, 132

hives, 124

hunger, sudden, 34, 46,

hyperactivity, 59, 95, 97, 141, 143, 181, 187

hypoglycemia, definition of, 45-46, 120

hypoglycemia questionnaire, 173-174

hypothyroidism, 138

I

inner trembling, 46, 121, 174

insomnia, 46, 94-95, 109, 114, 174

insulin, 45-46, 111-112, 114-115, 122-123, 126, 133, 136, 141, 143-144

J

juvenile delinquency, 40-41, 59

L

lactose, 58

Larson, Dr. Joan Mathews, 107, 109, 127, 130-132, 176

learning difficulties, 59, 181

Lee, Leslie, 20, 152, 169

M

Ma Huang, 141

massage therapy, 73, 85

medication, 30, 35-38, 48-49, 56-57, 59, 62, 67-70, 73, 95-96, 102, 115, 128-129, 139, 143, 144-145

Mendelsohn, Dr. Robert S., 47

mental confusion, 46, 104

menstruation, 68

mood swings, 46, 52, 92, 94, 113, 126, 128

muscle/joint pain, 57, 73, 85

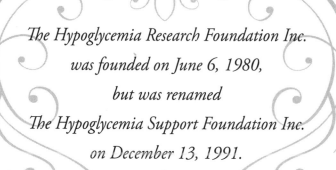

The Hypoglycemia Research Foundation Inc.
was founded on June 6, 1980,
but was renamed
The Hypoglycemia Support Foundation Inc.
on December 13, 1991.

"I considered myself to be s a strong and healthy 28 year old man. I worked hard, exercised extensively and thought I had the world on a string! It all caught up with me! The extra hours, junk food, coffee and extra-strong, energy drinks put my body in such a state; I thought I was going to die! I wound up in the ER. Thank goodness it turned out my blood sugar; the doctors said it was extremely low, in the 40's. I had no idea what that meant. Luckily my girlfriend Googled low blood sugar and found your website. From there we purchased your book. It was life-altering! At first I thought I could do this, just change my eating habits. Then realized, after reading every chapter, I needed more. Slowly but surely, I made changes—one step forward and one step backwards. It all paid off! It's been one year now and my energy has almost retuned, I'm back at work, exercising but not to extent. Most of all my eating habits have changed. My motivation—I was too young to go through life living like I was old and sick. You and your book were an inspiration to me… I am forever indebted!"

Paul—Queens Village, New York

"I just found your website, www.hypoglycemia.org and Facebook page. Then I immediately went out and bought your book. I can't tell you how much I appreciate all your information and support. It is so comforting to feel I am not alone! My only regret is not taking this path sooner."

Cecile—Houston, Texas

"I have been sick for over 12 years. Never associated my symptoms with what I was eating or drinking. It wasn't until I went out with some friends that one of them said she had a severe case of hypoglycemia. After describing her symptoms, diagnosis and treatment; I knew immediately I had to find out if this was my problem. Low and behold, I was confirmed by my chiropractor! I got a copy of your book and between my doctor's advice and the suggestions in your book — I'm on the road to recover — after all these years! Why did I wait so long! "

Marilyn—Kansas, Missouri

" I don't hide it, I am an alcoholic! I've tried everything I could for the past 20 plus years to kill this "devil" in me! I actually gave up hope that I would find an answer or a cure. Then I accidentally came across your book. It was on the table in a friend's house that I was visiting. While he was in the kitchen, I picked it up and browsed through the pages, came across the chapter on the correlation between Hypoglycemia & Alcoholism and stopped in my tracks. I asked to borrow the book, came home and read it. It transformed my life! I still have a long way to go but realize now that unless I change my eating habits, there's little chance of recovery. The sugar and caffeine have to go! I've been encouraged to reach out for help. Without your book and my new direction, I have no idea where I would be today!"

Glenn—Pensacola, Florida